To our friend,
Sebastian,
whose vision
birthed this book,
and whose daring brought
books about cannabis
and other entheogens
to independent minds
around the world.
Thank you, Sebastian.
We miss you
and your good works.

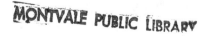

Other Books By Dr. Beverly Potter

Overcoming Job Burnout: How To Renew Enthusiasm For Work

Finding A Path With A Heart: How To Go From Burnout To Bliss

The Worrywart's Companion: 21 Ways to Soothe Yourself And Worry Smart

From Conflict To Cooperation: How To Mediate A Dispute

Brain Boosters: Foods & Drugs That Make You Smarter

Drug Testing At Work: A Guide For Employers And Employees

The Way Of The Ronin: Riding The Waves Of Change At Work

Turning Around: Keys To Motivation And Productivity

Preventing Job Burnout: A Workbook

Other Books By Dan Joy

Better Sex Through Chemistry: A Guide To The New Prosexual Drugs & Nutrients

The Healing Magic
Of Cannabis

DR. BEVERLY POTTER
DAN JOY

RONIN PUBLISHING

POST OFFICE BOX 1035

BERKELEY, CA 94701

THE HEALING MAGIC OF CANNABIS
ISBN: 1-57951-001-9
Copyright 1998 by Beverly A. Potter

Published and Distributed by:
RONIN PUBLISHING, INC.
Post Office Box 1035
Berkeley, CA 94701
www.roninpub.com

Project Editor:	*Sebastian Orfali*
Developmental Editor:	*Beverly Potter*
Manuscript Editor:	*Dan Joy*
Copy Editor:	*Nancy Freedom*
Cover Design:	*Brian Groppe*

ACKNOWLEDGMENTS

We thank those who spent time reading passages of *The Healing Magic of Cannabis* as the manuscript was being developed and appreciate the thoughtful feedback from Graham Bonnar, Markus Hawkins, Linda Lawrence, Cate Leggett, Galen Newman, and Simone 3rd Arm. Well-deserved gratitude goes to Erik Linden, who provided important material, tireless administrative assistance, and much good cheer during the project's early stages. When technical questions arose regarding psychopharmacology or chemistry, we were extraordinarily fortunate to have access to the world-class expertise of Alexander Shulgin, Ph.D. We were lucky to have Nancy Freedom available for timely delivery of thorough copy-editing. We are especially grateful to the ever-present Tucker the Talker, who provided the crucial canine perspective on the issues addressed in this book and proved that a dog is truly a writer's best friend. Lastly, our heartfelt appreciation goes out to you, dear reader, with our sincere hopes that *The Healing Magic of Cannabis* brings healing magic into your life.

NOTICE TO READER

Information presented in this book is made available under the First Amendment of the Constitution. It is a general overview of medicinal cannabis and should not be considered medical advice. The publisher and authors do not claim medical authority. Always consult your doctor or other qualified health practitioner before using cannabis medicinally. The publisher and authors do not advocate breaking the law. Medical marijuana has been legalized in certain states through voter initiatives. The reader should realize, however, that even in areas where initiatives for medicinal use of cannabis have passed into state or local law and even when the cannabis has been purchased from a cannabis buyers club, the purchase and consumption of that cannabis may still be a crime under federal law. Individuals wishing to use medicinal cannabis should consult an attorney about its status in their area before doing so.

TABLE OF CONTENTS

INTRODUCTION

Cannabis has been used by human beings around the world for medicinal, nutritional, recreational, spiritual, and industrial purposes for thousands of years. This book focuses on the specifically medicinal or healing uses of cannabis. The word "cannabis", for the purposes of this book, refers to strains of the plant whose leaves and flowering tops contain active concentrations of this herb's sixty-plus unique medicinal and psychoactive compounds, called *cannabinoids*, the most widely acknowledged of which is delta-9-tetrahydrocannabinol, or THC. Not at issue here are the stems of the plant from which fibers are obtained for industry and craft, the roots of the plant which are toxic, the seeds of the plant which have nutritional value, and strains of the plant that have industrial or other value but are not psychoactively or medicinally potent.

WHAT IS HEALING?

Healing is often somewhat erroneously equated with medical cure. The concept of healing, however, includes but is broader than that of cure. Cure is a physical phenomenon, whereas healing can occur on any or all levels of a person's being—body, mind, and spirit. Healing—which may or may not encompass physical cure—is the process of positive, empowering, and progressive reconciliation and transformation in a person's relationship to his or her reality, condition, history, and circumstance, inclusive of any diseases. When it comes to disease conditions specifically, healing refers to positive change in the impact of disease on a person's life, feelings, consciousness, decisions, and actions. In healing, a person's experience of disease, and the effects of disease on the body and mind, change for the better, whether or not physical cure is affected.

Healing, therefore, can take many forms. It can include making peace with oneself, one's past, family and friends. It may manifest in better relationships or a more peaceful acceptance of a disease condition—whatever restores balance and harmony to one's life. Healing can occur through an effect as simple, although powerfully, as the easing of pain. Pain relief can bring forth profound transformation in the effects a disease has on a person's outlook and abilities to enjoy life, connect with others, and achieve.

HOW CANNABIS HEALS

Cannabis, as far as we know, does not operate as a cure *per se* for any particular physical condition. The spectrum of ways through which cannabis can serve as an agent of *healing*, however, is vast and varied, encompassing an enormous range of disease conditions. Cannabis can relieve pain where other drugs or techniques have failed, opening the door to all of the healing benefits and increased life options of pain relief. Through its soothing and enlivening mental effects, the psychoactivity of cannabis can by itself be extraordinarily healing, cleansing the outlook and renewing enthusiasm for life. Cannabis also has direct, beneficial physiological impacts on certain diseases such as glaucoma, migraine, multiple sclerosis, and epilepsy. These positive physiological effects, while less than "cure," are certainly healing properties.

This description highlights the three basic channels through which cannabis serves healing. These are: 1) palliative, the overall soothing and the easing of pain; 2) psychoactive, or changes in state of mind; and 3) biological, the direct interference with disease processes on a physiological level. The nature of these categories and the interactions between them will be explored in the section of this book dealing with specific medical conditions.

HEALING AS A RE-CREATIONAL ACTIVITY

The concept of healing used in this book is broad enough to encompass the notion of truly recreational activity. The original meaning of the word "recreation," after all, refers to transformation, or re-creation, to "creating again". *Truly* recreational activity, then, is regenerative, life-giving, transformative—in other words, healing. So when cannabis is used in a genuinely recreational capacity, such usage is a form of healing. And the well-directed medicinal use of cannabis is also healing—in other words, transformative, regenerative, or re-creative. The word "healing" thus points toward what both medicinal *and* recreational use of cannabis *can* be, at their very best. By focusing on the process of healing, then, this book bridges and unites the recreational and medicinal approaches to the use of cannabis. The notion of healing, referring to positive transformation on the level of spirit as well as body and mind, also encompasses the *entheogenic*—spiritual or religious—approach to the use of cannabis.

HEALING AND TERMINAL ILLNESS

Healing can happen even in the face of death. For instance, healing can occur in the context of an apparently irreversible terminal condition through arrival at a deeper acceptance of death, dissipating the fear and denial that surround death, enhancing enjoyment, appreciation, and positive use of precious remaining days and hours, and increasing communion and intimacy with others to warm the last hours of life.

Psychologist Dr. Timothy Leary, a pioneering researcher into the positive potentials of psychoactive and entheogenic substances such as cannabis, provided a remarkably colorful and potent demonstration of a healing approach to dying during his final months. He emphasized the awe, mystery, and excitement available through facing the adventure of dying directly, and invited millions through the media and possibly hundreds through personal visits to share in his celebration of this experience. The principles behind his dying process—which was most certainly assisted by psychoactive medicines, including cannabis—were described in his final book, *Design for Dying*, co-written with R.U. Sirius.

Cannabis can serve as a remarkable agent of healing for dying people, easing pain and fear of death, enhancing appreciation and enjoyment of the present moment, engendering a more spiritual attitude toward death, and encouraging conviviality with loved ones and caretakers. William B. O'Shaughnessy, M.D., a 19th Century pioneer of the medical use of cannabis, referred to the healing in the face of death that the plant afforded his patients as "strewing the path to the grave with flowers."

WHAT IS MAGIC?

The sense of the word "magic" used in this book bears reference neither to sleight-of-hand trickery, nor specifically to the use of occult or sorcery technology such as charms, spells, and incantations. *Webster's New World Dictionary of American English, Third College Edition* offers some more relevant definitions: "any mysterious, seemingly inexplicable, or extraordinary power or quality" and, quite simply, "producing extraordinary results, as if by magic or supernatural means." Thus, the phrase "healing magic of cannabis" refers to the extraordinary power or quality of cannabis as a tool for healing, and to the extraordinary results that can be achieved through its use in this capacity.

The phrase "healing magic of cannabis" also bears deeper additional meanings. Occultists define magic as change or transformation affected in accordance with personal will. A classic symbol for this transformation is the alchemist's conversion of lead into gold. This transformation can occur in the arena of the material world—for instance, the body—or in the realm of consciousness. It is well-known that cannabis can be used to make desired consciousness changes possible information is achieving increasingly widespread dissemination, that the use of cannabis can also bring about desirable changes in the body in certain disease state as described in Part Two of this book.

According to the definition of magic as bringing about desired (or willed) change or transformation, healing magic can be considered the process of bringing about desired healing changes or transformations. The "healing magic of cannabis," therefore, refers to the extraordinary, "magically" powerful results that can be achieved by the use of cannabis as a tool for unlocking the healing power of the mind.

BODY, MIND, AND SPIRIT

In the ancient Chinese Taoist philosophy, healing, magic, and spirituality were inseparable. Similarly, the ancient Sumerians, whose geo-cultural is considered "the cradle of civilization" (and who used cannabis in the practice of divination), saw no separation between these three fields of human understanding and endeavor. This book, while based on modern medicine and psychology, brings this kind of ancient, integrative understanding to bear on its subject matter. This is an understanding in which spirit, magic, and healing are united. This book applies such understanding in a practical way to the medicinal and healing use of cannabis, discussing how cannabis can be employed as a medicine for the body, mind, and spirit.

PSYCHOACTIVITY CAN HEAL

The psychoactivity of cannabis is a major asset to its ability to promote healing. Findings in the field of mind/body medicine reveal that positive changes in mental state can have an enormous healing impact on the physiological level. Elevation of mood—the promotion of optimistic outlook accompanied by relaxation and the blossoming of hope, faith, and humor—is the central fountain from which the healing potential of cannabis' psychoactivity springs. Through its psychoactive properties, cannabis can ease tension, reduce stress, elicit relaxation, and foster optimistic thinking and positive mental attitudes. It can empower healing visualization practices, strengthen faith, and promote humor and laughter. All these qualities of mind support the body's natural inclination toward wellness.

WHO CAN BENEFIT FROM THIS BOOK

The Healing Magic of Cannabis is addressed to two categories of people. First are those who want know if and how cannabis can be useful for their medical condition or that of a patient or loved one. Second are those already using cannabis for healing purposes who seek to deepen their understanding of how their medicine works and desire to maximize its positive potential. Most particularly, this book intends to help those using cannabis medicinally to amplify those changes in consciousness that can catalyze and facilitate the physical healing process. Even though the learning process by which a person comes to navigate, channel, and manage the mind-changes facilitated by cannabis is usually intuitive, occurring largely outside of conscious awareness, it can nonetheless be brought into consciousness. Then it can be directed and amplified by conscious will, focus, intention, and discipline. This process can be thought of as a form of magic—bringing about desired change through application of will.

By no means does The Healing Magic of Cannabis intend to recommend cannabis for everyone—not even everyone who suffers from one of the conditions for which cannabis can be useful. No book or treatment regimen can fully account for the precious uniqueness, the singular individuality of body, mind, and spirit, that is evident among all human beings. No medicine is for everyone, and cannabis is no exception. In a culture where the approach to health is dominated by modern Western medicine, which often tends to gloss over individual differences as it seeks a reliable treatment for everyone (or nearly everyone) suffering from a particular condition, it can be easy to forget an important fact: The magic of healing is always performed by the unique bodies and minds of unique people. Appropriate treatment can vary as widely from person to person as much as people themselves differ. Therefore, a treatment that succeeds for one person may fail for another, no matter what that treatment is. A doctor or caregiver who is ideal for one person might be completely inappropriate for another, just as one person's well—chosen life partner would be a ruinous mismatch for another.

This book is meant to help readers make an informed decision as to whether to undertake integrating cannabis into their healing process, and to help them make the most positive use of cannabis if it is already a part of their regimen. If you use the material in this book, work with your doctor or other health practitioners to adapt the information to fit your personal situation. Take what it is discerned that you can make use of, and put the rest aside.

Always consult a doctor or other qualified health practitioner before adding cannabis to your treatment program. If the decision is made to use cannabis for healing purposes, do so with appropriate feedback and supervision. The ma*terial in this book is provided to inform and should never replace the supervision of a physician or other licensed health practitioner.*

PREVIEW

The first several chapters of *The Healing Magic of Cannabis* explore the healing potential of cannabis' psychoactivity. This part of the book begins with a brief summary of recent findings in mind/body medicine, a field devoted to the role of states of mind in health, illness, and healing. The next chapter gives an overview of the nature and characteristics of cannabis' mental effects, highlighting potentially health-promoting qualities and offering special focus on how the plant's psychoactivity can be employed for relief of pain. Each of the four chapters that follow investigates a specific property of the plant's psychoactivity. The properties focused upon are relaxation, humor, optimism, and spiritual faith. Each chapter reviews medical research linking the quality of mind or state of consciousness under discussion to health, immunity, and recovery from disease. Furthermore, each of these chapters offers material of practical value for channeling, directing, and deepening specific mental effects of cannabis, suggesting ways by which the flexibility of mind engendered by the plant's use can be taken advantage of to achieve mental states conducive to health and immunity.

Part Two of *The Healing Magic Of Cannabis* shifts to a nuts-and-bolts focus on the preparation and use of the plant for medicinal purposes, covering all of the known routes by which cannabis can be administered medicinally, their advantages and disadvantages, and their relevance to specific disease conditions. Included are various standard means of smoking and inhalation, recipes for cannabis-containing foods, and procedures for preparing and using tinctures and topical applications of the plant.

The third section of *The Healing Magic of Cannabis* is specifically medicinal in orientation, beginning with an overview of the history of the plant's medical employment, its physical and physiological effects, and its medicinal chemistry. Then goes on to cover in depth a wide range of the medical conditions that cannabis can be used to treat, discussing each condition, how cannabis acts to relieve it through the interplay of palliative, psychoactive, and biological healing effects, and appropriate administration.

The closing chapter of The Healing Magic of Cannabis takes a brief but practical look at the distinction between use and abuse of this medicinal plant and attempts to glimpse what new developments the future might hold for the healing application of cannabis and its derivatives.

Cannabis aside, this book is a reminder of the healing power of hope, faith, optimism, serenity, and humor. These are the mental conditions that liberate and empower the body to perform its own mysterious and astonishing healing magic. Even more magical than cannabis' many palliative and biological properties is this plant's ability to help people tap into these enormous healing resources of the mind and spirit.

PART ONE

CHAPTER 1

THE HEALING MIND

Positive mental states like faith, optimism, courage, serenity, and good humor exert profound influences on physiology and immunity, helping us to stay well and to overcome challenging illness. Conversely, negative emotions like depression, pessimism, and conflict contribute to the development of health problems and impede recovery from disease.

THE HEALING MIND

In recent years physician writers have popularized mind/body medicine, which focuses on the ways that psychological and spiritual states like thought, emotion, belief, and faith affect health and recovery from disease. There is an increasing interest in the roles of psychological states and spiritual experiences in health, disease, and recovery. Mind/body medicine integrates the use of guided imagery, trance, hypnosis, and other consciousness-altering techniques—even prayer—into individualized treatment programs, usually in conjunction with conventional medical practices.

In his book, *Spontaneous Healing: How to Discover and Enhance Your Body's Natural Ability to Maintain and Heal Itself*, Andrew Weil, M.D., relates the stories of people who have healed from severe illness in a seemingly miraculous fashion—even though doctors told them they had no chance of recovering. Many recoveries took place without the medical interventions doctors had insisted were the only hope of survival. Weil says spontaneous healing is a frequent occurrence, not a rarity, and that it usually occurs after a breakthrough change of mental state.

While healing *can* happen without any profound change of heart or mind, the mind is nonetheless a crucial trigger of the healing system. Activating the mind through a mental shift is a key to engaging the healing processes.

The well-known *placebo effect* serves as a potent demonstration of the mind's healing power. The phrase "placebo effect" refers to patients who get better after taking a placebo, from an injection or a pill that contains no medicine, and is attributed to the patients' positive expectations that the therapy will work.

The placebo effect proves that the mind has formidable capabilities once thought to belong only to the realm of magical powers wielded by wizards and sorcerors. Like the fabled sorceror-alchemists of old, who turned lead into gold, the mind has the power to transmute an inert substance, such as a sugar pill containing no medicine, into a healing agent.

THE HEALING POWER OF MIND-CHANGE

The yearning to alter consciousness is a necessary, fundamental, and instinctual desire. In his book on drugs and higher consciousness, *The Natural Mind,* Weil argues that wanting to alter consciousness is an innate, normal drive similar to hunger or the desire for sex.

Enjoyment of periodic non-ordinary consciousness is demonstrated by children who are far too young to have learned it from social influences. Toddlers the world over, for instance, often whirl themselves like beginner dervishes until they achieve a dizzy stupor. Babies or young children will sometimes sit or stand and stare fixedly at some object for a long time, which is a standard technique for inducing trance states. The fact that such mind-altering behaviors appear so universally among the very young points towards the innate, perhaps even biological, nature of the human drive to change states of consciousness.

Propensity to alter consciousness is an important key to physical, mental, and spiritual health. Altered states characterized by deep relaxation, for example, are associated with physiological benefits that help us stay well and fight disease. The heightened awareness brought about by physical activity such as "runners' high", is part of what draws people to integrate healthy exercise into their lifestyles. Altered states can be used to help bring about desired psychological and behavioral change. And the urge to change awareness fuels our spiritual aspirations, leading us towards prayer, meditation, and other forms of contemplation. These examples just begin to hint at the broad range of physical, psychological, and spiritual benefits to be gleaned from entering alternative states of awareness.

Mind-altering drugs have been used since primitive times to satisfy the human appetite for altered consciousness. Cannabis, for instance, is the only crop ever to have been cultivated by the Pygmy tribes of Africa. Their folklore holds that the Pygmies' relationship with the mind-altering plant goes back to the dawn of time. For centuries the "mystery religions" around the Mediterranean carried out a days-long ceremony of initiation involving intense alterations of consciousness, including the ingestion of a secret elixir that almost certainly included psychedelic ingredients. Socrates, Aristotle, Plato, and Hippocrates were initiated into the Mysteries, and made awed references in their writings to the rites' life-changing power.

Dismissing as errant activity the use of cannabis and other psychoactive substances is to deny its historical and cultural ubiquity. Weil, among others, argues persuasively that drugs—intelligently used as tools to enter other states of consciousness—can be beneficial.

THE FOURTH DRIVE

Research psychopharmacologist and UCLA professor Dr. Ronald K. Siegel unfolds a similar argument in his book *Intoxication*. Like Weil, Siegel links the use of drugs to alter consciousness to an instinctual drive—only Siegel goes a step further. He holds that the use of psychoactive substances is not just *one form* through which this instinctive urge can be expressed; rather, the urge to alter one's consciousness with drugs is *itself* a "fourth drive," on a par with the drives to eat, drink, and have sex. Like these other drives, the fourth drive is a characteristic human beings share with other members of the animal kingdom. For instance, strung-out horses "steal" the toxic *locoweed*, a hallucinogenic plant native to the American Southwest, whenever they get a chance. Toward the close of his book, Siegel boldly states that our need for intoxicants is natural, even healthy.

CANNABIS' PSYCHOACTIVITY

Psychoactive drugs have value because they provide gateways to altered states. Cannabis is a psychoactive plant, and the altered state it brings about can facilitate healing. In fact, the cannabis' psychoactivity underlies much of its outstanding performance as a healing agent.

Cannabis helps create a mental shift that awakens the body's healing systems, the kind of mind-change that Weil points to as the key to healing. Cannabis promotes relaxation, and elevates mood through stimulating optimism. Cannabis tends to engender a more detached perspective on life, one of the main goals of spiritual practice, and is used by many to help inspire and stimulate spiritual faith.

Not only are such mental changes enjoyable in themselves, but they are good for immunity and physical health as well. The healing potentials and qualities of the cannabis "high" can be cultivated, deepened, and amplified through meditative practices, visualization, and ritual. All of these are consciousness-altering techniques that can be combined with the psychoactivity of cannabis to increase its mental and spiritual benefits, thereby magnifying the healing energies unleashed.

CHAPTER 2

PSYCHOACTIVITY AS A MAGIC HEALER

Cannabis is a *euphorigenic* plant which means it can generate euphoria in people who use it. The prefix *eu* in "euphoria" is the Greek word for "well," as in wellness. Thus, *euphoria* means "a state of well-being." This word, so commonly used to describe the psychoactive effects of cannabis, refers to the state of wellness the plant can help us to remember and thus help guide us back towards health.

The euphoria engendered by cannabis blends relaxation, light-heartedness, optimism, and a sense of safety. Mental stresses, worries, and concerns recede into the background, giving way to feelings of insight, wonder, pleasure in social contact, delight in simple things, and attention to the enjoyments available here and now.

EUPHORIA HEALS

Feelings of well-being are a primary quality of the plant's psychoactivity—its action upon the mind, or *psyche*—for most of the people who use it. So nearly universal is this response that the phrase "feels good when stoned" emerged in psychologist Dr. Charles Tart's survey on the effects of cannabis as one of the characteristic experiences associated with being high. Because feeling good—or feeling *well*—facilitates healing and maintaining health, the euphoria stimulated by cannabis, a very safe, non-addictive therapeutic substance, offers a healing opportunity unencumbered by the toxicity, complications, and perils connected to the use of many other euphorigenic substances.

ENHANCED SENSES

Perhaps the most notable and celebrated aspect of the cannabis high is enhancement of the senses. As the psychoactive effects unfold, every perceptual field becomes enriched as the details and subtleties within it are clarified and magnified. Colors, and the contrasts and complementarities between them, become brighter and more vivid. Sounds acquire greater depth, texture, and dimension, and the spatial and harmonic relations between them become more pronounced, leading to absorbed fascination with music.

Analogies for the difference between the senses unassisted by cannabis and the senses under the sway of its effects might be the difference in image between the washed-out picture on an old, defective television as compared to the brilliant colors and sharp resolution on a set you've just purchased, or the difference in the sound of music coming from a portable hand-held radio as opposed to a component stereo system. This sensory enhancement results in marked amplification of aesthetic sensitivity, deepened enjoyment of both natural beauty and works of art, and appreciation of details in the immediate environment that might usually be taken for granted or pass unnotice.

INTENSIFIED PHYSICAL AWARENESS

The psychoactivity of cannabis promotes a keener awareness of bodily states, physical sensations, and physiological processes that are normally ignored. Heightened somatic sensitivity might draw attention to breath, heartbeat, digestive processes, or subtle physical discomforts or minute muscular tensions that have been overlooked. It can increase the pleasure derived from stretching, exercise, or yoga, from the relaxation and comfort felt in moments of repose, and can even infuse with joy an act as simple as breathing.

DETACHMENT

Cannabis' psychoactivity engenders a detached, distanced point of view that allows a person to observe emotions, thought processes, sensations, and desires with a sense of neutral objectivity. While emotions and other sensations may be perceived with greater clarity and vividness, their grip on one's state of mind is lessened by a shift in perspective. In this state of letting go it becomes easier to disentangle oneself from the unrelenting obsession, compulsive cogitation, and shortsighted viewpoint that characterize our usual attachment to issues of concern. This quality of mind bears kinship with the state of detachment or objective "witness consciousness" cultivated and encouraged in many spiritual practices and traditions, such as the meditative disciplines of Zen Buddhism and the release of karma in Hinduism.

EXPANDED TIME

Cannabis brings about a distinct alteration in one's sense of time, which seems to proceed more slowly. A few minutes may feel like an hour; an hour may feel like two or three. In a fascinating study, Stanford University social psychologist Dr. Phil Zimbardo discovered that when hypnotized subjects were given suggestions that time was expanded, they acted much like a person experiencing a cannabis high. They became childlike, playful, and full of spontaneous laughter. Apparently there is something that psychologists don't yet understand about an expanded sense of time which enables us to lighten up, laugh, and feel good.

OPEN-MINDEDNESS

The psychoactive effects of cannabis facilitate the cognitive process psychologists call "free association," allowing one thought to lead to another and yet another in a series of links that are more novel and unpredictable than in the usual course of thought. In synergy with the detached perspective that infuses the cannabis high, this increased fluidity of thought leads many people to feel that their problem-solving capacities are enhanced, permitting them to conceive innovative solutions that otherwise wouldn't occur to them due to their rigid habitual ways of thinking. This mental loosening also permeates the creative process; many artists use cannabis for fresh inspiration.

HOW PSYCHOACTIVITY PROMOTES HEALING

Many aspects of the psychoactivity of cannabis foster healing. Among these are optimistic outlook, aesthetic enhancement, a sense of communion with others, body awareness, empowered imagination, increased feelings of control over one's state of mind and one's life in general, appreciation of the moment, and inspiration of transcendental experience.

OPTIMISTIC OUTLOOK

Fluidity of mental processes and optimistic viewpoint can help people form new perspectives on their illness and overall situation, leading them to contemplate and enact new strategies for dealing with problems, discomforts, and inconveniences. Their minds may become open to new, different, and possibly more effective possibilities of treatment. Additionally, optimism and positive belief have been shown to support health and bolster chances of recovery from illness.

AESTHETIC ENHANCEMENT

Enhanced sensory acuity can lead to immersion in appreciation of nature and works of art. Such moments provide pleasant distraction from pain and discomfort, making the course of an uncomfortable disease process easier to endure. It is also likely that such states of enchantment involve the release of endorphins and other neurochemicals that facilitate immunity and physiological healing.

COMMUNION AND COMMUNITY

People tend to use cannabis with friends, finding both that sharing the state of being high increases its pleasure and that it encourages sharing itself. Scientific research has confirmed that people who frequently engage in positive contact and communication with supportive others tend to be healthier and stand a better chance of recovery from serious illness.

LAUGHTER

The cannabis high is well-known for promoting humor and laughter. The sense of humor is one of the mind's foremost healing resources. Humor heals the mind by refreshing perspective and keeping our viewpoint balanced; it heals the body by inspiring laughter. The biochemical and physiological benefits of intense and sustained laughter—such as that which often accompanies getting high—are being revealed by medical research to be covered later in this book. Because stress and illness often challenge and compromise the sense of humor and the ability to laugh, the capability of cannabis to renew these faculties is an especially important healing asset for those combating a disease.

BODY AWARENESS

Enhanced perception of bodily sensations and physiological processes, combined with the sense of detachment that can make pain or other unpleasant sensations easier to examine with objectivity, can help a person to be more responsive to changes in physical condition, positive or negative. For example, a person might realize the need to practice deep breathing, make dietary changes, or to release muscle tension. Heightened bodily awareness might help a person to be more aware of small signs of improvement, thus fueling the optimism that quickens the healing process.

EMPOWERED IMAGINATION

The use of cannabis is classically associated with imaginative reverie, the "Technicolor daydream." This is because psychoactivity affords enhanced capacity to visualize and imagine—at length, in depth, and in detail. This quality can be harnessed to increase the intensity and impact of visualization and relaxation techniques used to engage the powers of the mind in healing.

GREATER SENSE OF CONTROL

Using cannabis to alter mood, outlook, and awareness, as well as to ease pain or other symptoms, can give people a sense of greater control over their state of mind and lives. Scientific experiments have shown that people with a greater sense of control over their circumstances and treatment stand a better chance of recovery from illness. This psychological factor appears to play a significant role in how well the immune system functions.

TRANSCENDENTAL EXPERIENCE

Cannabis has been used as a sacrament in religious rites of many traditions. The high promotes meditative stillness and contemplative awe and can give rise to religious experiences and feelings of spiritual faith. Cannabis has played a catalytic role in many profound transformative experiences that have people to embrace spiritual and meditative disciplines. Studies have shown that religious devotion and spiritual lifestyle are associated with good health and longevity, and that people strong in faith are more likely to be healthy and to recover from serious illness.

APPRECIATION OF THE MOMENT

How many times have we all wished for more hours in the course of a day? In a way, the time-expanding quality of the cannabis high bestows this gift of extra time, filling it with small beauties and delights, sprinkling the day with opportunities to "stop and smell the flowers" and encouraging us to live more fully in the here and now. Whether or not this property is of physiological benefit in the healing process, it is nonetheless a tremendous boon to the quality of life of those who are seriously ill.

Smell The Flowers

The Seeker and the Shaman Woman were sitting in a garden on a beautiful day when the Shaman Woman noticed that the Seeker was frowning and staring distractedly into the distance. "Is something troubling you?" asked the Shaman Woman.

"How can I enjoy my life when I know that sooner or later I'm going to die?" the Seeker lamented.

As the Shaman Woman listened she leaned over, picked a nearby lilac sprig and passed it slowly by the Seeker's nose. "Ah," the Seeker sighed, his frown dissolving into a smile.

"Humm," the Shaman nodded, "always remember to stop and smell the flowers."

GETTING HIGH IS LEARNED

As dramatic as the various features of the high may seem to be, the psychoactivity of cannabis is nonetheless a remarkably subtle phenomenon. Many people using it for the first few times claim not to be high and say they notice no effects. New users are often coached or "tuned into" the high by old-timers. In this sense, getting high has to be *learned*. And in certain ways this learning process can continue along with the continuation of a person's use of cannabis.

For instance, reverse tolerance means that as users become more experienced with the cannabis' psychoactivity, they require smaller amounts to achieve the same level or intensity of high. This aspect of cannabis' psychoactivity is probably largely a matter of a subliminal learning process. Using cannabis over time, a person learns about the states of mind and changes in mood that it facilitates. Once these mental territories have become familiar and mappedout, opening internal doors to them becomes second nature and it takes smaller amounts of cannabis to enter them.

DIFFERENT MINDS, DIFFERENT HIGHS

At different times, for different people, and with different strains of cannabis, the nature of the psychoactivity will vary. Some of the qualities described will predominate in certain instances, while at other times they may not be experienced at all.

The high is shaped by many factors. One is the chemical constitution of the cannabis being used. Cannabis contains approximately sixty therapeutically active compounds, many having some psychoactive effect. Those which are psychoactive vary in of their mental effects, and different strains of the plant feature different levels and proportions of these substances. Furthermore, the substances present in cannabis act in synergy and combination. For instance, CBD, a cannabinoid not generally considered to be psychoactive in itself, has been shown to moderate the psychoactivity of THC. Thus, the ratio of CBD to THC present in a given sample of the plant will figure in the nature of its psychoactivity.

Unique Responses

Another important shaping factor in the variable nature of pychoactivity is individuality, the uniqueness of every human body and mind. Some people report absolutely *no* psychoactive effect from cannabis, even some of those who use the plant consistently for painkilling and other medicinal purposes. And some people experience effects that are *opposite* to those usually described. For example, although relaxation is a typical response to ingesting cannabis, some people experience anxiety when they use it. For these people, obviously, use of the plant may be a less viable treatment option than for those who find cannabis relaxing.

How an individual experiences the psychoactivity of cannabis may vary with the passage of time. For example, some people who disliked the high during youthful experimentation have tried the plant again after a lapse of several years and found it quite favorable. Such variance occurs in conjunction with changes in biochemistry, mental state, and other conditions. Such changes in the nature of the plant's mental effects can serve as guideposts for an individual as to how, and whether, he or she can make use of cannabis at a given time. In general, the more favorable a person finds the mental effects of cannabis, the more likely it is to be of medicinal value for that person.

DOSAGE, SET AND SETTING

The nature of psychoactivity varies even more widely between different individuals and different occasions than the medicinal and other effects of non-psychoactive substances. In research at Harvard University in the early 1960s by psychologist Dr. Timothy Leary and colleagues, "dosage, set, and setting" were found to be primary factors in shaping a person's response to psychoactive substances. "Dosage" refers to the amount of substance consumed. "Set" refers to the mind state of the person who uses the substance. Current mood and preoccupations, and most importantly, beliefs and expectations regarding what the experience will be like, have a tremendous influence on the nature of any session with a psychoactive agent. "Setting" refers to the physical and interpersonal environment in which the person experiences the high.

The variable nature of psychoactivity reminds us that the act of getting high is performed by the mind, not by the substance. While the substance is a stimulus, the high itself is the mind's *response* to that stimulus. This process is analogous to healing. Treatments don't heal; minds and bodies heal, with the assistance of treatments.

USING PSYCHOACTIVITY TO HEAL

Because a person's mind plays such a formative role in the nature of psychoactive effects, one can use knowledge, intuition, inspiration, experience, judgment, and desire—all properties of the mind—to guide and shape the nature of the changes in consciousness ones experiences with cannabis, just as a sculptor shapes a piece of clay into a work of art.

Working with altered states of consciousness in this way, like piloting a boat, is a skill that can be learned and refined over time. For the person using cannabis for healing purposes, there can be great rewards in engaging in a conscious, directed learning process regarding the potentials of its psychoactive properties. No matter how familiar one may already be with cannabis' mental effects, one can still learn even more about working with its psychoactive effects to derive optimal value from the healing opportunities offered. Opening doors to alternative states of awareness and directing the energies so released along pathways that lead toward wellness is a skill that has been practiced and taught by specialists in healing from ancient to present times. Examples include tribal shamans, modern hypnotherapists, and contemporary doctors who practice a mind/body/spirit or holistic approach to medicine.

As experience with cannabis' psychoactivity grows, a person can learn to take increasingly skillful advantage of the flexibility of mental state that it catalyzes. Using as a basis the favorable "take-off weather" that cannabis offers, awareness and attention can be refocused and piloted with increasing surety and steadfastness into positive healing states that are ever deeper, more complete, and more beneficial.

USING PSYCHOACTIVITY TO CONTROL PAIN

Altering one's state of consciousness can have remarkable results in the relief of pain. Hypnotherapy, the induction of trance states for healing purposes, has a history of amazing successes in this area. Sometimes the skillful use of hypnosis and trance can make severe pain disappear from a person's awareness entirely, at least for the period of the trance in question. The use of hypnosis to control pain during childbirth has become widely accepted, even in hospitals.

Although not all of the cannabinoids that demonstrate significant painkilling or analgesic properties have psychoactive effects, the alteration of consciousness induced by cannabis nonetheless plays an important role in the overall soothing of pain and general easing of physical discomfort that the plant offers. Working with the psychoactive component of cannabis' pain-relieving properties is a good example of how the plant's mental effects can be directed and amplified for healing purposes.

PSYCHOACTIVITY CREATES DISTANCE FROM PAIN

As the euphoria associated with cannabis flourishes, the plant's uplifting impact on mood and the positive thoughts and feelings that accompany it tend to take the sufferer's mind off the pain. While the pain may still be present, it fades into the background as the mind focuses on more positive alternatives and other subjects, thoughts, and sensations. A shift occurs in perspective regarding the pain and how it is perceived in relation to overall experience. This alteration of perception as it takes place in mind is a psychoactive effect.

This experience has been described as the pain slowly receding into the distance, as the clanging sound of a loud gong ringing on the beach would fade into the background for a person on a boat floating away from the shore. To take this metaphor a bit further, when the boat puts down anchor and stops at a certain distance from the beach, the person on the boat can still hear the gong. Perhaps he or she can even still hear it quite clearly and distinctly; but it's no longer loud, overwhelming, and unpleasant, dominating awareness. The person can concentrate on other sounds, pulling them into the foreground and perhaps forgetting about the sound of the gong entirely.

When the perspective regarding the place of the pain in overall awareness has shifted, the mentally soothing effects of cannabis facilitate a gentle redirection of attention towards things of beauty that give joy and pleasure. For the person on the boat, these might be the soothing sound of the lapping ocean waves or the graceful arcs traced by the wings of seagulls in flight above. These aesthetically pleasing sensations and beauty give rise to optimistic thoughts and feelings of hope and faith.

While cannabis may be the "boat," providing a means of transportation to this state of euphoria, the healing shift of consciousness is not automatic. It is accomplished by the mind. Cannabis serves as a tool of the mind that increases the flexibility of its state, loosening it from its attachment to pain and the negative thoughts arising from it.

Cannabis is like a solvent applied to the paint on a canvas, softening the hardened colors, unsticking them from the surface, making them fluid again allowing one to pick up a paintbrush and change the picture—one's state of mind.

REFRAMING ALTERS PERCEPTION

A shift into a more positive state of consciousness can alter the experience of pain. A key to the transition into optimistic modes of thought and positive beliefs is a phenomenon called *reframing*. In reframing, which is a shift in perspective, the role that a negative factor plays in a person's thinking, perceptions, and beliefs changes. Saying that a glass is half full instead of half empty is an example of reframing. The glass remains the same while what you pay attention to about the glass changes.

When the context in which a problem is seen changes, it has been put into a new "frame"—a different set of beliefs about, and ways of looking at the issue. With those beliefs come expectations about what's going on and what will happen. Expectations shape our lives because we tend to make our expectations come true. When our "picture" is put into a new frame, things look different and we respond differently to them. Reframing is one form of transformative healing magic. As we transform our outlook, our quality of life and ability to heal also become positively transformed.

Reframing of negative situations can lead to the negative factor becoming merely *less* negative. One example of such reframing is when pain fades into the remote background, allowing focus on other thoughts and sensations.

In a more complete kind of reframing, a formerly negative factor actually becomes *positive*. For example, when viewed from the point of view or frame created by pessimism and fear-based thinking, getting fired from a job is a loss, a cause of fear and worry, perhaps even a disaster. A person in such a situation who has managed successfully reframe this life circumstance, however, could look at the situation as a chance to get some needed rest and relaxation, review their options, and pursue a more fulfilling form of employment. Another example of reframing that most people have experienced is that of listening to the roar of a freeway. This sound can be annoying and stressful, especially if it is coming from outside your bedroom window when you're trying to sleep. However, if you tell yourself that the noise is the sound of a rushing river, it starts to sound like it really is a river. Whereas moments before it may have been aggravating, the same sound becomes soothing and actually helps you fall asleep.

Reframing requires mental work. It doesn't happen automatically: it may take some creative thinking, followed by persistent and persuasive self-convincing, to come to see in a positive light a factor or situation that initially appeared, unfortunate or burdensome. The altered state of cannabis, and the partial reframing of pain that it induces, can be used to facilitate this kind of complete reframing.

REFRAMING PAIN WITH PSYCHOACTIVITY

One way to lessen pain through reframing is to *externalize* it. The heightening of imagination and sense of detachment promoted by cannabis can be used to help visualize the pain as if it were located *outside the body.* The pain can be projected into an external imaginary or real object, like a block of wood or a stone. A common meditative exercise to externalize pain involves standing or sitting on the ground, preferably in a pleasing natural setting, and projecting the pain down into the ground, letting it be absorbed and soothed by the healing Mother Earth.

Another externalizing technique is to imagine a duplicate of your own body, or some other imaginary body, and imagine that the pain is occurring in the corresponding part of *that* body and that *your* body does *not* hurt in that place. This technique reframes the pain by making the pain no longer *your* pain, but instead *a* pain in *another* body.

Mental redefinition, or reframing, of this sort has been used by people to enable them to endure extreme feats of self-imposed pain such as those performed by Far Eastern fakirs who, among other impressive demonstrations of pain control, can sit or lie for long periods of time on a bed of nails. A man who had studied firewalking demonstrated what he learned by walking barefoot back and forth on broken glass. Amazingly, he did not cut his feet. He explained he imagined that he was walking in a refreshing stream and what he felt under his feet was pebbles on the stream-bed, not broken glass. The power of the mind is so great, and the power of our ability to reframe perception—is so magical that this man was unharmed.

The psychoactivity of cannabis has many features that can be put to use in the service of healing. Bringing these features and their healing potential into conscious awareness and working with them actively and intentionally can increase their healing value. Using mental reframing techniques to build on the distance from pain that the psychoactivity of cannabis provides is one way to amplify a healing property of cannabis' mental effects through directed effort. Later chapters in this book will provide techniques maximizing cannabis' ability to promote relaxation, humor, and even spiritual faith—all healing properties.

Psychoactivity is in many ways like a key that can open doorways to healing. While cannabis may provide us with this key, in order to take full advantage of psychoactivity's healing potential we must make the effort of using the key to unlock the door.

CHAPTER 3

CANNABIS MELLOWS

It's no coincidence that the word "mellow" is a synonym for the experience of a good cannabis high. Many people use cannabis primarily for its ability to relax them, making it a key component of cannabis' healing magic, with benefits to body, mind, and spirit.

RELAXATION AS A MAGIC HEALER

Relaxation is a wellspring from which many of cannabis' other healing benefits flow. The mental relaxation facilitated by cannabis soothes the worried mind, softens the hardened, pessimistic outlook, and engenders a flexible, optimistic, and hopeful viewpoint that aids healing. Relaxation restores humor, allowing the recovery of perspective and the release of tension through laughter that eases suffering and bolsters immunity. On the spiritual level, relaxation provides the soil in which the state of consciousness known as "quiet mind" can take root. From the quiet mind emanates spiritual faith, a tremendous resource for healing that soothes the body and fuels recovery from disease.

STRESS KILLS

Some studies indicate that stress is a factor in as much as eighty per cent of physical disease. Emotional stress has been shown to accelerate the spread of cancer. High stress levels push the body into a state of alert called the fight-or-flight response, which temporarily shuts down certain immune functions in order to maximize the physiological resources available for grappling with the stressful situation at hand.

Chronic stress generates a kind of physiological "noise" causing us not to hear significant bodily cues—signals as simple as the rumblings of the stomach that tell us it's time to eat, or small pains that inform us of an injury or might indicate a condition that could become worse. The voice of the body becomes lost in the din.

RELAXING IS HEALTHY

Relaxation is the antidote to stress. Relaxation is marked physiologically by an increase in slow brain waves and decreases in metabolism, blood pressure, heart rate, and breathing rates. Harvard Medical School professor Herbert Benson, M.D., trained patients to enter the deep relaxation he called "the relaxation response" by focusing the mind on the silent, internal repetition of a chosen word or phrase for ten or twenty minutes a day while gently brushing aside intruding thoughts— a method similar to prayer and traditional yogic mantra meditation. Relaxation can also be elicited by activities as varied as gazing at sunsets and certain kinds of rhythmic body motion.

Benson's work demonstrated that regular practice of relaxation combats hypertension, helps with cardiac arrhythmias, decreases pain levels, reduces PMS symptoms, and assists in sleeping. He says that when the relaxation response occurs, "your mind and body suddenly become a five-star resort in which all the service personnel make your restoration and health their priority and are especially concerned with alleviating the harmful effects of stress."

People with AIDS who practice relaxation have fewer symptoms, and cancer patients experience similar benefits while having fewer problems with reactions of nausea and vomiting to chemotherapy. Regular practice of relaxation increases self-esteem while reducing anxiety, depression, and anger. Cannabis' ability to reduce stress and promote relaxation, without severe side effects or interference with normal physiological and mental function—unlike most other antistress medications— underlies a great deal of its medicinal value.

REMEMBERED WELLNESS

In his book *Timeless Healing,* Benson attributes the body's ability to heal to "remembered wellness." He asserts that "all of us have the ability to remember the calm and confidence associated with health and happiness, not just in an emotional or psychologically soothing way; this memory is also physical." The memory of being well—an inner knowledge and understanding of vitality and wholeness, of what it means and how it feels to truly thrive—is woven into the fiber of our being, all the way down to the cellular level. It is this template of health that guides the process of healing. Like a lighthouse on the horizon guiding a ship back to port, this deep, bodily recall of the condition of well-being is the beacon upon which the body fixes its sights in order to navigate its way from illness back to health.

RETURN TO BALANCE

The human body is a *homeostatic* organism, one which strives to maintain equilibrium through ongoing adjustments in its physiological processes. Remembered wellness is the blueprint of equilibrium, providing guidelines for the physiological adjustments that allow return to balance from illness. The body's natural tendency is to maintain health, regaining equilibrium when external influences have shifted it out of balance. However, homeostasis can be obstructed when barriers to the memory of wellness develop, like ocean mists gathering to obscure the helmsman's view of the lighthouse beacon from the shoreline.

Foremost among barriers to remembered wellness is stress, which fosters rigidity locking conditions of illness into place. Relaxation, which Benson identifies as a primary key to the activation of remembered wellness, dissolves the barriers of stress that occlude the cellular memory of health.

Tod Mikuriya, M.D., a leading champion of the medicinal use of cannabis, observed that, in addition to the relaxation it promotes, it can assist in the recall of forgotten memories. Through relaxation, awakening of lost memory, and its other effects, cannabis for many people rekindles *feelings* of wellness, helping both our bodies and minds to recall what it is to be whole. Leonard, a middle-aged cancer patient undergoing chemotherapy who used cannabis for nausea and loss of appetite, describes how cannabis-induced relaxation vividly brought forth forgotten, happy memories of his youth. Not only did Leonard *remember* the feelings of being healthy, vital, whole, and strong when young; it was as if these feelings actually *returned*, if only for a few moments at a time, to his afflicted body. These episodes of remembered wellness vastly improved his spirits and, he felt, furthered his restoration to health.

RELAXING WITH CANNABIS

Generally, people don't realize they are tense and don't know how to relax. For most of us, therefore, relaxation is like any other skill: it must be learned. Cannabis can assist. Using the plant reliably promotes a physical relaxation in which the mind remains alert. States of this kind are ideal for learning in general, and particularly for learning to relax.

Central to the skill of muscular relaxation is the ability to recognize subtle physiological sensations of tension when they occur, especially in its beginning stages, when the tension is still at a low level and is thus easier to release.

By amplifying and thus helping us to tune into this level of minute sensation, cannabis' psychoactivity can be of particular help in learning relaxation. Sharon, herbalist and student of yoga, finds this quality of cannabis so compelling that she likes to perform ten or fifteen minutes of yoga stretches as soon as the soothing effects and increased bodily sensitivity begin to set in, selecting postures specifically suited to release the previously unnoticed areas of muscular tension.

Studies show different levels of benefit depending on how long and how often relaxation states are maintained. Allowing yourself to "hang out" in a relaxed state for ten to twenty minutes (once or twice a day) will help generate maximum benefits.

TENSING AND RELAXING THE MUSCLE GROUPS

Learning to relax involves recognizing and detecting tension by comparing sensations of tension with those of relaxation. With practice, one can detect finer and finer gradations of sensation associated with increasingly subtle levels of tension. Doing this can be accomplished through the practice of systematically tensing and then relaxing specific muscles, while comparing the feelings produced.

Practice Often

The enhanced awareness of subtle sensation promoted by cannabis can facilitate learning how to relax. By learning to self-induce and release increasingly minute levels of tension and recognizing the feelings so created, one becomes capable of detecting and releasing increasingly subtle muscular tension throughout the body, thereby preventing it from building into a painful rigidity that is more difficult to release. When tension is noticed in, for example, the neck, one can focus attention upon it, take a deep breath, and then willfully release neck tension.

Regular practice of tensing and relaxing various muscle groups in a given sequence helps in maintaining a more relaxed overall muscle tone as well as in becoming familiar with the sensations of tension and relaxation as they manifest in specific body areas. The use of cannabis can facilitate the learning process that this discipline stimulates by intensifying and therefore making it easier to observe, remember, and compare the sensations associated with tension and relaxation in each muscle group.

This simple relaxation practice can be performed by tensing and relaxing a muscle or muscle cluster, one at a time. With the eyes closed, the specified muscle is tightened in conjunction with a long, slow intake of breath. Care should be taken not to tighten the muscle too much, but just enough so the tension is noticeable. Study the physical sensation of tension in that particular muscle while maintaining the tension for a count of seven (except in the case of the feet, where tension should be maintained only for a count of three to avoid cramping). Then quickly release the tension as much as possible from the muscle in conjunction with a deep, complete exhalation. Study the sensation of relaxation for ten or more seconds. Repeat this process of tensing and relaxing muscles one by one until you've practiced with all muscle groups.

MUSCLE GROUPS AND HOW TO TENSE THEM

Arms and Hands
• Hand and forearm: Make a fist.
• Biceps: Bend arm at the elbow and make a "he-man" muscle.

Face and Neck
• Face: Squint, wrinkle nose, and try to pull entire face into a point at the center.
• Forehead: Knit or raise eyebrows.
• Cheeks: While clenching the teeth, pull corners of your mouth towards your ears.
• Nose and upper lip: With mouth slightly open, slowly bring upper lip down to lower lip.
• Mouth: Bring lips together into a tight point, then press mouth into teeth. Blow out gently to relax.
• Mouth: Press right corner of mouth into teeth and push corner slowly toward the center of mouth. Repeat for the left corner.
• Lips and tongue: With teeth slightly apart press lips together and push tongue into roof of mouth.
• Chin: With arms crossed over chest, stick chin out and turn it slowly as far as it will go to the left. Repeat for right side.
• Neck: Push chin into chest at the same time as pushing head backward to create a counterforce.

Lower Body
• Buttocks: Tighten buttocks and push into chair.
• Thighs: Straighten leg and tighten thigh muscles.
• Calves: Point toes towards head.
• Toes: Curl toes under.

BREATHE DEEPLY TO RELAX

Slow, steady, smooth, deep breathing immediately elicits relaxation. Unfortunately, many people breathe shallowly, which keeps old air in the lungs, preventing them from getting filled completely with new air. Shallow breathing contributes to muscular tension.

During inhalation the diaphragm, the layer of muscle located between the lungs and the abdomen, contracts and descends, increasing lung capacity. During exhalation, the diaphragm relaxes and moves upward, forcing the air out. Therefore, with full, complete breathing, the abdomen should expand outward upon inhalation and withdraw inward upon exhalation. Correct breathing can be checked by placing the hand on the abdomen and seeing if it moves outward with inhalation and inward with exhalation.

How To Breathe Deeply

To develop skill at breathing fully and regularly, and to create a daily relaxation break during which the body can rest and repair, the following exercise can be performed for five to ten minutes each day. Using cannabis beforehand can help in slowing down and focusing attention on the process and sensation of breathing, thereby deepening relaxation and accelerating learning.

> **Step 1:** Inhale slowly for four seconds; hold the breath in for four seconds; exhale slowly for four seconds; hold the lungs empty for four seconds.

> **Step 2:** Mentally count the breaths from one to four as follows. As you inhale, count "one." For the moment that you hold the breath in, think "and." Then, as you exhale, count "two." Think "and" to count the moment that the lungs are held empty. For the next inhalation, count "three." Think "and" to mark the hold phase, and exhale with a mental count of "four," thinking "and" while holding. Then begin again with inhaling for a count of "one."

> **Step 3:** Focus all your attention on breathing and counting.

Hold your hand on your abdomen the first couple of times you perform this exercise to make sure you are breathing correctly. As you gain skill and lung capacity, slowly increase the length of time taken for each phase first to a count of six, then to a count of eight. When you find your attention wandering, gently let go of distracting thoughts and return your attention counting.

COUNTDOWN TO RELAXATION

Counting backwards while imagining yourself descending stairs is a technique often used in hypnosis because it is an easy way to achieve a state of mental and physical relaxation. Using cannabis in conjunction with this exercise can potentiate its benefits because of cannabis' ability to relax the body while keeping the mind alert.

The counting method beings with picking a spot twenty to forty-five degrees above eye level and staring at it until the eyelids start to feel heavy, then letting them close gently. For unknown reasons, pointing the eyes slightly upward with the eyes closed in this fashion stimulates the production of alpha brainwaves, which are associated with deep relaxation. The next step is to imagine yourself slowly, steadily descending a long flight of stair while mentally counting backwards from 100 to one, spacing the counts at intervals of about two seconds apiece.

Most people become reasonably relaxed the first time they perform this technique. Skill at rapidly entering increasingly deeper relaxation can be built by practicing the method daily while "condensing" it over time. For the first ten mornings, perform the exercise by counting backward from 100 to one. For the second ten days, count backward from fifty to one. For the third ten-day period, count backwards from twenty-five to one. For the fourth ten-day period, count backward from ten to one. At the end of forty days of such practice, most people can achieve deep relaxation just by looking upward, closing their eyes and counting backward from ten to one.

DEBRIEFING

Deep relaxation is usually concluded with a "debriefing" phase for gently returning to the here and now to smooth the transition back into the waking state.

Before debriefing, allow yourself time to remain in a state of deep relaxation, breathing slowly and deeply while keeping your eyes closed.

Notice how you feel. Acknowledge and enjoy any feelings of wellness and sensations of enlivening, healing energy coursing through your body. The effects of cannabis tend to make such sensations more vivid and intense, and thus more easily noticed and deeply appreciated. Allow these positive sensations to continue in your awareness while you sit quietly with eyes closed for a few more moments.

When ready, count slowly from one to five, allowing about two seconds for each count. While doing so, imagine yourself going upstairs to return to a waking state. When you have finished, open your eyes and affirm to yourself that you feel good and are wide awake and ready to resume activities.

REMEMBER YOUR WELLNESS

Recalled and imagined sensations are more intense when a person is deeply relaxed. For instance, when one in a waking state is asked to imagine swimming, a simple mental image, an abstract image or *concept* of swimming is likely to come to mind. By comparison, when a person who imagines swimming when deeply relaxed is likely to actually *feel* sensations of swimming, like the pressure and feeling of water on the limbs and skin, the taste of water in the mouth, and the sound of splashing. Relaxation empowers the imagination to create an intensity of sensation akin to that of dreaming. This phenomenon explains why relaxation techniques are invariably an integral part of imagery techniques or *autogenic* visualizations, such as those used by cancer specialists Carl Simonton, M.D., and Stephanie Simonton, used to treat disease and promote health.

Like relaxation, and no doubt at least in part due to its relaxing qualities, cannabis also imparts vividness and depth to imagined and remembered realities. The psychoactivity of cannabis in tandem with the power of relaxation provides an especially powerful combination for intentionally calling forth vivid memories of wellness. Immersing oneself in their detailed recollection has a soothing, vitalizing, and enlivening effect, and may in fact open a bridge to the cellular blueprint of health that Benson identifies as the basis of all healing.

IDENTIFY TIMES OF WELLNESS

In order to intentionally activate the phenomenon of remembered wellness, begin by thinking back across your life, scanning your memory for times when you felt especially whole, well and vibrant. Relax and take your time performing this review, allowing yourself to enjoy each memory at a leisurely pace.

Then select one memory to focus on in particular. Use the counting backward technique to enter deep relaxation. When you feel deeply relaxed, recall the time of wellness as vividly as you can. Imagine yourself being back in that time and place, observing the world as you saw it then. Notice what is there, taking the time to savor each detail. Check in with all five of your senses. What do you see? What sounds do you hear? What do you smell? What do you feel? Can you taste anything? Concentrate particularly on *bodily memory*, how it feels to have a body that is strong, well, and alive with energy, and allow yourself to fully enjoy reliving sensations of well-being. When ready, bring your attention back to the present.

An elderly professor who uses cannabis to ease the pain and inflammation accompanying arthritis remembered a hike he took in his early twenties through an aspen forest in Colorado. This memory was particularly appropriate because it recalled the strength, endurance, and resilience of his young joints and muscles before his arthritis set in, as well as the scenes of natural beauty to which this physical hardiness allowed him access through the long, strenuous hikes he had so enjoyed. He noticed the cool, crisp air scented with ocha roots, the gray-white branches reaching to the sky, and the golden sunlight filtering through the aspen leaves.

Regularly repeat the practice of recollecting a chosen time or times of wellness. The detail and vividness of the experience—and therefore its potential healing power—deepens with each repetition. This process can be facilitated by keeping a journal in which you record details and impressions after each visualization. To stimulate memory and provide a basis for further recollection, the notes in your journal can be reviewed before each practice.

Times of wellness usually share a common quality: that of a deep and confident calm and relaxation. This is a reminder of the fundamental role of relaxation in health and healing and helps explain why relaxing can elicit memories of wellness.

TAMING THE MIND FOR RELAXATION

Unwelcome, and troubling thoughts can interject themselves and distract us even when we are deeply relaxed. It's easy enough to latch onto these thoughts, which inevitably lead to further thoughts and the interruption of our relaxation. *Resisting* these thoughts, however, is just as distracting, and just as disruptive to relaxation, as the thoughts themselves.

The Mind Is Like A Wild Elephant

"Shaman Woman, when I try to quiet my mind, it runs on and on wildly," the Seeker complained. "The harder I try to hold it back, the more unruly it gets."

The Shaman Woman nodded sympathetically, "Your mind is like a wild elephant. When you try to control it, the elephant will resist by rearing up, flapping its ears and roaring as it tries to run free."

"Then what can I do?" asked the Seeker. "How can I tame my wild mind?"

"Don't scold the elephant when it runs," the Shaman replied. "Instead, gently but firmly pull the it back. Again and again the elephant will run, and again and again you must pull it back. Eventually, the elephant will know you are the master. Then you can use its great power. The same is true of your wild mind."

It takes practice and a great deal of patience to tame your wild mind. Intrusion of irrelevant thoughts does not represent failure at this endeavor; rather, it is to be expected. Letting go of internal mental chatter is an integral part of learning deep relaxation.

When mental noise intrudes into your practice, simply notice the intrusive thoughts dispassionately, without criticizing yourself for their occurrence. Then just let them go—*effortlessly,* as if you were simply setting something down to leave it on the side of the road as you walk along. Gently return your attention to the object of your mental focus, whether it's counting backwards, an internal image, or a mind-quieting device such as the repetition of a word, phrase, or rhythmic body movement.

Strive to maintain a passive attitude toward mental chatter. Simply notice the interruption and then return your attention to your practice. Remember that *getting frustrated* about interruptive thoughts is itself destructive to mental quiet.

RELAXATION PROMOTES HEALTH

Relaxation is a crucial health skill, restoring calm and balance to our bodies and minds, dissipating the barriers of stress that block our pathway to wellness. Most of us have become so acclimated to stress and tension that we must learn, or at least re-learn, how to relax. Cannabis, relaxation techniques, and soothing visualizations are all powerful methods for educating ourselves in the art of relaxation, and they are especially effective when combined. The disciplined and focused use of cannabis along with relaxation and visualization can help bring about a less stressed baseline condition of body and mind, allowing us to go about the pursuits of daily life in a more relaxed condition that permits deeper rest and sleep, promotes overall health, quickens recovery from illness, and makes all of our activities more enjoyable and rewarding.

CHAPTER 4

CANNABIS IS UPLIFTING

*B*elief is a fundamental force in healing. Such is the power of belief that it plays a critical determining role in whether a medical treatment succeeds or fails, and sometimes it is sufficient to bring about cure in the absence of any treatment at all.

All disease is psychosomatic. This is not to say that the mind is responsible for all disease—as the term is commonly misunderstood—but rather that disease always has both physical and mental components, affecting and being in turn affected by processes occurring in body and mind. This is true of even the simplest and most harmless of conditions. At the center of the mental component of illness is belief. This is the main mental factor determining of what course disease will take.

The kind of beliefs at issue in illness and health take the form of expectations, optimistic or pessimsitic. We expect relief, improvement, and eventual wellness, or we expect continuing ill health and decline.

Oncologists Carl Simonton, M.D., and Stephanie Simonton studied cancer patients with spontaneous remissions—people who got better without any medical explanation. They found that people who defied medical statistics had something in common: a positive, optimistic and determined attitude. In fact, the entire spectrum of inquiry into the relationship between mental states and physical health, from surveys and rigorous scientific experiments to the testimonies of shamans and faith healers, continually reaffirms a simple truth: optimism heals. It promotes maintenance of good health as well as more rapid, complete and sometimes even "miraculous" recovery. Conversely, pessimism afflicts. It diminishes vitality, increases the frequency and duration of illness, and in some instances wields fatal power.

CANNABIS PROMOTES OPTIMISM

The psychoactivity of cannabis strikes to the core of the mental component of disease by encouraging optimism. Cannabis engenders appreciation of the present moment and encourages the belief that a brighter destiny will unfold. By loosening our attachment to habitual thinking patterns, cannabis empowers us to challenge pessimistic thoughts and to explore more hopeful paths of thinking. By opening the mind to new alternatives, cannabis combats feelings of helplessness and gloom that accompany disease and immobilize the will. Use of this beneficial plant can thus help restore belief in our capacity to shape our own destinies—increasing the chances that, through both belief and action, we will do so.

BELIEF CAN HEAL OR HARM

Beliefs determine how the world looks to us. The present that is perceived, the past that is remembered, and the future that is imagined, are all images shaped, textured, and colored by beliefs. Most importantly, beliefs dictate how we respond to the present, and so inform the future that we create for ourselves; and as it turns out, this principle operates not only in behavior but in physiology, down to the level of cellular immune activity. The quantities of chemicals released by our glands, the vigor with which our cells battle pathogens, the tenacity and resilience of our tissues, and other physiological processes are tempered and empowered—or dampened—by what we believe. Our beliefs, therefore, play a clear role in scripting the future of our bodies.

A 1950 study investigating the relationship between belief and healing produced astounding results. Pregnant women suffering from severe nausea and vomiting were given a drug usually used to *induce* vomiting, and were told it would *cure* their nausea. Amazingly, they *all* stopped vomiting and being sick to their stomachs—*completely*. Through the power of the expectation that the medicine they were using would make them better, they healed themselves—and in doing so, their minds managed to completely reverse, or at least neutralize, the medicine's usual effects.

PLACEBO EFFECT

These results can be explained by the *placebo effect*, a phenomenon first reported in 1945 that has formatively influenced the methods by which medical research has been conducted ever since. The placebo effect refers to the observation that positive medical results will be reported among a significant percentage of patients who have not been given an actual medication but instead a "dummy" pill or injection (a placebo) containing no active substances. The power of the placebo is attributed to the patient's *belief* that the medication is effective. Recent research indicates that the placebo effect is vastly more powerful than originally estimated.

In *Timeless Healing: The Power and Biology of Belief,* Harvard Medical School professor Herbert Benson, M.D., identifies three belief-related factors that figure in the outcome of a treatment. First, is patients' beliefs and expectations regarding the treatment outcome. Second, is beliefs and expectations on the part of health practitioners and personal caretakers. Third, is beliefs and expectations generated in relationships between caregivers and patients. These influences are so important that Andrew Weil, M.D., who has been in the forefront of research into the mind's role in healing, maintains that belief, in both practitioner and patient, is *the crucial factor* in determining a treatment's success or failure.

SELF-FULFILLING PROPHECIES

Just *how* positive expectations work to promote physical healing is a mystery. Apparently immune and regenerative activity, as well as other physiological processes, respond to beliefs—specifically, beliefs that bear on health, beliefs about whether we will recover and become well, whether the treatment we are using will work, whether our doctor is a good one—almost as if they were commands. In response to these messages, our bodies work towards fulfilling the prophecies of our beliefs.

The good news here is that *our beliefs are not set in stone*, but are more transitory, more malleable than one might think. Certain aspects of belief shift quite readily and frequently,   undergoing changes that usually occur outside of conscious awareness.

Flexibility of belief is reflected in our changes of mood and outlook. The beliefs from which we are operating in any moment change along with our mood and state of mind. Sometimes, we have an optimistic, can-do frame of mind. When we're in such a mood, we operate and respond on the basis of belief in a positive future where we have the power to influence things in the direction of our desires. When in a pessimistic mood, on the other hand, we tend to operate from the belief that the future will likely be negative no matter what we say or do.

The Simontons, whose research was mentioned earlier, made positive use of this malleability of outlook. They demonstrated that visualization and other techniques for developing positive mental attitude can achieve remarkable results in controlling cancer spread and growth.

Because our moods and states of mind can be altered through practices ranging from meditation to recreation, so can the beliefs with which they are associated. We can enhance health and help to weight the outcome of physiological processes in favor of future wellness by cultivating optimistic mood-states that send positive belief messages to our cells and organs.

OPTIMISM THROUGH PSYCHOACTIVITY

The healing power of the mental messages we send our bodies can be enhanced by the use of substances that act upon the psyche to unleash its capacity for generating moods and mind-states that promote optimism and health. While it is the mind that generates such states, psychoactive agents can *activate* the mind's capacity to do so. For most people, cannabis functions with remarkable speed and efficacy in just this way.

Furthermore, cannabis is a mood-positive psychoactive presenting a minimum of possible side effects, health hazards, and complications, especially as compared to those presented by other available mood-altering substances, including standardly used pharmaceutical antidepressants that are considered "safe". For instance, while cocaine might momentarily promote a can-do attitude, it taxes the body and depletes the biochemical systems associated with positive moods. Therefore, cocaine and similar psychoactives are unlikely to be used to any ultimately health-enhancing effect. Cannabis, however, in addition to its positive palliative and biological benefits in regard to various physical conditions, is not known to present such complications.

KEY CHARACTERISTICS OF OPTIMISM

To understand how cannabis can assist in the cultivation of optimistic outlook, it helps to look at the components of optimism, and those of pessimism, its "evil twin" counterpart. Through such an examination we can see how specific qualities of cannabis' psychoactivity correspond to key characteristics of optimistic thought processes while counteracting pessimism. Our exploration will focus on two essential components of optimistic outlook: habitual disputing of negative thoughts and belief in the individual's power to take charge of personal circumstance and destiny. Cannabis' mental effects relate specifically to these cornerstones of optimism. Having these properties of the cannabis high brought to our attention can help us amplify the assistance in breaking free of pessimistic thought and action that the plant's psychoactivity offers us.

DISPUTING PESSIMISTIC THOUGHTS

One of the cardinal characteristics of pessimism is the ongoing occurrence of negative thoughts. This pattern is so automatic and ingrained in those prone to pessimistic states that such thoughts appear and accumulate in the mind usually without even being noticed, let alone questioned, by the person who thinks them.

A cardinal characteristic of optimism, on the other hand, is disputing negative thoughts as they occur. Whereas a pessimist will instantly formulate and unquestioningly accept a negative conclusion about a situation, an optimist will notice and critically examine such an assessment for flaws. When a pessimistic judgment is revealed as invalid by internal disputing, the optimist will replace it with a more positive—and more reasonable—re-evaluation. Optimism thus requires consideration and creativity, while pessimism is a distinctly rote, predictable style of thinking.

Cannabis is well-known for its long association with a critical, questioning approach to ideas promoted by traditional and cultural authority. The plant also encourages the questioning and disputation of one's *own* thoughts and beliefs. This property works against the automatic, mechanical nature of pessimistic thinking, and thereby assists in cultivating optimism—a more creative way of thinking.

Detachment

Two aspects of cannabis' effects on cognition work together to make the examination and disputation of automatic thought processes both easier to perform and more likely to happen in the first place. The first of these is mental detachment. The detached point of view towards one's own thought and feelings that is engendered by cannabis allows a person to observe them as if from a distance, with a sense of neutral objectivity. The usual grip of automatic thoughts on the state of mind is relaxed by a shift in perspective. In this state of consciousness it becomes easier to disentangle from the unrelenting obsession, compulsive cogitation, and shortsighted viewpoint that characterize pessimism.

Most of us pay little attention to our own thought processes. This is particularly so for habitually pessimistic thinkers, in whose minds negative assessments and conclusions are reached with automatic rapidity. Often, all that is consciously perceived is the negative conclusion, which is accepted without awareness of the automatized thinking processes upon which it is based. In order to dispute thoughts, one has to observe them in the first place. The detachment facilitated by cannabis promotes just this kind of self-observation.

Expanded Time

The second aspect of cannabis' mental effects that facilitates disputing one's thoughts is the sense of expanded time. As mentioned, pessimistic thought processes tend to occur so quickly has a chance to observe, let alone dispute, the nature of the thinking involved. The steps in thinking and the links between them pass by too rapidly to be seen or questioned.

With the assistance, however, of the expanded time-sense promoted by cannabis, it becomes easier to observe the stages of thinking as they take place. The slowing down of the time-sense creates an effect like playing back a videotape of the thought process at slow speed, allowing events and details that would normally be missed to become evident. It's as if the "train of thought" becomes an actual train passing before the mind's eye. The engine, caboose, and cars between—the components and stages of the thought process—are each available to be noticed and inspected. Their value, accuracy, and appropriateness, and whether they really belong in the "train" at all, can be contemplated. The integrity and strength, or lack thereof, of the links between the cars— the soundness of one's logic—also becomes more evident. Furthermore, the uplifting nature of cannabis tends to lead this process of evaluating and reconstructing one's thought processes towards conclusions more optimistic and hopeful than those reached through rote, automatized pessimistic thinking.

With conscious awareness of the facets of cannabis' psychoactivity that aid in observing and disputing pessimistic thought processes, one can increase the advantage they offer, employing them purposefully to develop skill in combating pessimism and promoting optimism in one's thoughts. In doing so, one can promote health and help to activate healing energies in the body.

CAN-DO ATTITUDE

Alongside disputing negative thoughts is a second key characterisitc of optimism: a determined, resilient, "can-do" attitude. This aspect views "negative" aspects of a situation as challenging opportunities to bring about change. It recognizes that many such "negatives" are in fact subject to change, and that at least many such changes can be effected by the optimist himself, who believes himself capable of changing whatever can be changed.

It's not hard to see how this aspect of optimism can assist healing in the most straightforward, practical, concrete ways. After all, a person with this kind of attitude is much more likely to research, choose, seek out, and follow through with an effective treatment program, performing whatever activities and making whatever commitments that are that patient's responsibility, as well as supplementing with additional health-enhancing practices of their own choosing.

In *An Alternative Medicine Definitive Guide to Cancer,* Robert C. Atkins, M.D., says a cancer patient's survival is based less on the severity of the disease than on the patient's attitude. He stresses the importance of patients resisting the intimidation and gloomy prognoses characteristic of orthodox medicine and taking active, assertive roles in their own healing processes. Atkins claims that having a "fighting spirit" is *the most important psychological component* for promoting survival of cancer.

Battles are won or lost because of mental attitude according to Fredrick Lovret, author of *The Way And The Power: Secrets of Japanese Strategy.* The deciding factor on the battle field is *kokoro,* "heart," the mental attitude of the warrior. Samurai knew honing a fighting spirit is essential to winning with the sword. The same is true in the battle against cancer and other diseases. Fighting spirit is built from intention, impeccability, and ruthlessness. John-Roger in *Spiritual Warrior* describes impeccability as an internal discipline of acting purposefully—maintaining a focus on the mission (which in this case is healing) even in the face of emotional crisis, illness and conflicts.

Roll The Joint Impeccably

The Shaman Woman and the Seeker were walking along a road when the Shaman stopped to roll a joint. Just then a speeding truck vered off the road right where the Shaman and the Seeker would have been if they had not stopped.

Shaken, the Seeker exclaimed, "Shaman Woman, if you hadn't stopped to roll a joint that truck would have hit us!"

"Yes, when we stopped we saved a moment and were not hit by the truck. But when walking along the road on another day we might lose a moment by stopping and then be hit by the truck."

"How can I know whether to stop or not to stop?" worried the Seeker, more agitated than before.
"You can't know," answered the Shaman. *"You can only
seek your quiet mind and roll the joint impeccably."*

Studies show that people who have a can-do sense of control over
the course of their lives are healthier than people who don't. In one study,
a broader range of daily lifestyle choices was offered to residents in one
wing of a facility housing elderly people than in the other wing. The
choices were simple, and seemingly rather trivial, like food menu items
and television programming. Sure enough, over the next several months,
those residing in the "freedom of choice" wing experienced significantly
fewer illnesses, and even fewer deaths, than those living in the wing
where matters like what would be served for lunch or shown on TV were
decided by the administration.

Once again, *belief* is at the core of the can-do attitude's healing
power. Researchers have determined that it's not the actual *range* of
options, but rather the belief that one has control over them, that makes
the difference in terms of health and illness. In other words, it's not how
much control one *really* has, but rather how much control one *believes*
one has, that sends a healing—or harming—message to the body.

HELPLESSNESS UNDERMINES HEALING

Just as a sense of personal potency enhances health, feelings of
helplessness can be utterly lethal. Feelings of helplessness, closely associated with a pessimistic outlook, send a dampening shut-down message to the body that tends to deactivate the healing process.

A pessimistic attitude—springing from the belief that the future is
bleak, and there's little or nothing one can do to change it—gives rise to
feelings of helplessness. Where there is no help, there is no hope; feelings
of helplessness thus give rise to depression, and the immobility with
regard to positive action and making decisions that accompanies depression.

Just as a can-do sense of optimism assists healing in simple,
practical ways through its motivating, energizing influence on personal

decisions and actions, a pessimistic sense of helplessness undermines healing. People depressed and immobilized by feelings of helplessness are less likely to follow through with their responsibilities in a treatment program, and are less likely to seek treatment in the first place. In his classic work, *Helplessness: On Depression, Development, and Death,* psychologist Dr. Martin Seligman shows that feelings of helplessness interfere with problem-solving, decision making, and other cognitive functions that can be crucial to survival for people in situations of life threatening illness.

Furthermore, chronic depression and the biochemical deficiencies associated with it undermine immune response on a biological level. In depressed people, infections tend to last longer. Feelings of helplessness may be instrumental in the formation of cardiac arrhythmias. Seligman's research has made it clear that for a person or animal in a weakened state due to aging or malnutrition, a sense of control or helplessness can make the difference between life and death.

Those already suffering from serious medical conditions are especially vulnerable to the waning of healing energies that follows on the heels of helpless thinking. Feelings of helplessness are often engendered by disease. Various levels and forms of physical immobility, and the need for assistance in carrying out routine daily tasks, are often consequent to physical disabilities that can accompany a wide range of conditions and disorders. Furthermore, the often authoritarian atmosphere of the conventional medical system, and the highly regulated, bureaucratic routines common in hospitals, treatment centers, and other "care" facilities tend to exacerbate this problem through enforced patient disempowerment.

These very specific, *real* forms of helplessness can trigger a downward spiral that is toxic to the healing process by encouraging belief in a more generalized personal helplessness. This kind of belief not only increases the suffering in enduring a disease but also sends signals to the body that ultimately undermine prospects of improvement, recovery—and restoration of personal autonomy.

People whose personal health and freedom are threatened by circumstances and physical conditions featuring a high propensity for this vicious cycle may stand to benefit from medicines that not only ease symptoms and combat disease physiologically, but offer help in reviving the sense of personal power. Cannabis appears to be just such a medicine.

FIGHTING SPIRIT

Fortunately, as Seligman's research shows, helplessness can be unlearned and optimism can be learned. Part of the value of biofeedback techniques, for instance, is the sense of empowerment that comes from learning that you can influence what goes on in your own body through exercise of will. Cannabis can also facilitate learning or re-learning a hopeful, empowered attitude about one's health.

For whatever reasons, cannabis has traditionally been associated with social, artistic, and political circles and subcultures placing a high value on novel, creative thought and personal empowerment. The controversial herb has been perennially used as both a vehicle of and a symbol for independence, individuality, autonomy, and the wresting back of control from traditional sources of authority. The questioning openness of mind released by the cannabis high seems to encourage people to re-evaluate what they do and don't have control over, what can and can't be done, and what endeavors are realistic and worthwhile or futile and naive. Furthermore, the plant's psychoactivity also seems to guide the process of questioning it initiates towards optimistic, often visionary conclusions about individual and collective possibility.

QUESTION AUTHORITY

Cannabis was virtually inseparable, for instance, from the grassroots movement that led the nation to question, re-evaluate, and ultimately bring to an end its involvement in the war in Vietnam. While polls and surveys showed after a certain point in time that most citizens (passively) opposed the war, it was a cannabis-fueled sociopolitical avant-garde who were optimistic and determined enough to believe that they actually had the power to *do* something about the issue. And to this end they tirelessly invented and enacted new, creative, and even bizarre forms of social action, from the antics of the Chicago Seven Trial to the levitation of the Pentagon. Is it any coincidence that hemp was smoked by George Washington and other fellows of the revolutionary cabal that founded our country by pulling off a maverick, unlikely rebellion based on idealistic principles?

The psychoactivity of cannabis, in sum, seems to promote just the kind of questioning, optimistic, can-do attitude and fighting spirit needed by an ailing person who is vulnerable to feeling trapped by the medical system and robbed of hope by statistical chances of recovery. Remarkable spirit and courage of this kind, in fact, has been brilliantly and consistently demonstrated by many often severely medically challenged movers and shakers in the grassroots medicinal marijuana movement, who have succeeded in changing laws and developing their own institutions as a result of their determination to return the power over their medical treatment into their own hands.

If psychoactivity awakens within the mind previously mired in feelings of helplessness even the merest glimmering of hope that control of destiny can be restored, quickening and enlivening messages of healing are sent to the cells and organs of the embattled body.

Beliefs and expectations are key forces in health and illness. It is as if, through beliefs and expectations, the mind either liberates or sets limits on the body's latent healing powers. Beliefs and expectations are aspects of mind, or consciousness. By bringing about alterations in consciousness, cannabis stimulates the kinds of beliefs and expectations that send empowering messages to the body and liberate healing energies.

CHAPTER 5

THE HEALING GIGGLE

The detached perspective engendered by cannabis opens our eyes to the humor and absurdity in the events and concerns that normally cause stress. This aspect of cannabis' psychoactivity incites us to laugh—sometimes uncontrollably! The well-known phenomenon of "the giggles" prompted Timothy Leary to joke that the only fatalities associated with cannabis over its millennia of usage were two people who "laughed themselves to death." This laughter-promoting quality is an important aspect of cannabis' healing magic.

LAUGHTER'S HEALING POWER

Norman Cousins, M.D., a famed explorer of the role of mental states in combating disease—especially cancer— emphasizes the power of laughter as a force for healing and recovery. He speaks from personal experience as well as extensive and original research in his book *Head First: The Biology of Hope*. Cousins survived a particularly debilitating and painful form of cancer in which he could barely move his arms and legs to turn over in bed, and his jaw was almost locked. In the midst of a situation that was anything but funny, Cousins laughed his way back to health by continuously watching Marx Brothers movies. He discovered that 10 minutes of genuine belly laughter had an anesthetic effect that enabled him to get a couple of hours of pain-free sleep—and was able to measure specific positive physiological changes that would occur after intense bouts of laughter. Cousins attributes his remarkable recovery to these massive self-administered infusions of humor.

Laughter heals. It promotes and strengthens communion with others, refreshes perspective to make it easier to deal with difficult situations, and even fosters health on a physical level.

CONVIVIALITY

Laughter is an agent of social connection and bonding. It relaxes and liberates, dissolving the defenses with which we keep others at a distance. When we laugh with others, we feel closer to them making the time we spend with them rewarding, and so motivating us to spend more time together. People who laugh together tend to stick together.

The interpersonal communion promoted by shared laughter is a healing force. Research shows that companionship, social support, and a sense of community are good for health. People who spend significant amounts of time in the company of supportive others get fewer diseases, heal faster, and live longer. By facilitating shared laughter, cannabis widens the doorway to the healing benefits of human bonding.

Cannabis also engenders a spirit of conviviality that leads to healing laughter. Laughter is fundamentally a social phenomenon. People laugh much more frequently when in the company of others than when alone, partly because of laughter's contagious nature. One person's laughter triggers another's in an effect that bounces back and forth like a ping-pong ball, extending and amplifying the laughter of each. Sometimes the laughter of just one person in a crowd triggers a ripple effect that cascades across the group until everyone is laughing.

People suffering from serious illness tend to withdraw and become reclusive, feeling self-conscious about their disease and that their condition may be burdensome to others. Cannabis lightens such heavy attitudes and promotes conviviality, making us more likely to seek the company of others. The use of cannabis therefore encourages people to avail themselves of the benefits to health afforded by both interpersonal engagement and the laughter that arises from it.

LAUGHTER REFRESHES PERSPECTIVE

We're all familiar with the psychological benefits of humor and laughter. The doctors and surgeons in the popular 1970's TV series

M*A*S*H* exemplified the importance of maintaining humor in the face of extraordinary stress and challenge. Much of the humor exchanged among its characters—and the laughter it provoked among its viewers—sometimes seemed inappropriate, even downright mean spirited, occurring as it did in the face of horrific tragedy, injury, and death. The point, however, was the power of humor to keep the characters sane, competent, and effective under these immense wartime pressures. By helping the members of the medical team to remain clear-headed, their humor literally saved lives. The promotion of humor—and therefore sanity—under such conditions was, no doubt, an underlying factor in the popularity of cannabis among American soldiers in Viet Nam.

Laughter functions as a release mechanism, triggering the catharsis of stored emotion, soothing tensions and easing anxiety and nervousness so that we regain balance and see matters in a fresh light, freeing the mind for problem-solving. Finding the humor in stressful situations helps one remain creative under pressure, work more effectively, and play more enthusiastically. The change in perspective brought forth by the cannabis "giggles" enables one to gain distance from ill health—if only for a moment—promoting positive feelings, helping us to become more resilient, creative, and optimistic and thus better able to handle the pressures that a healing crisis presents.

LAUGHTER HEALS THE BODY

The old adage that "laughter is the best medicine" is being confirmed by medical research. Laughter heals physically as well as psychologically. Intense laughter exercises the muscles of the heart, cleanses certain organs and tissues of toxins, and lowers blood pressure. Cousins' research showed that sustained laughter releases brain chemicals called endorphins, which reduce physical and psychological pain and boost immunity. Research at the Loma Linda School of Medicine showed that laughing activates the body's natural killer cells which fight pathogens and speed up the production of new immune cells.

A deep belly laugh is a physical workout. Stanford Medical School psychiatrist William Fry, Jr., M.D., who researched the physical effects of laughter, made an astounding observation. Twenty seconds of sustained laughter exercises the heart as much as three minutes of strenuous rowing. This assertion may seem far-fetched until you remember the last time you laughed so hard it actually hurt. You might have had to hold your stomach due to intense heaving of the diaphragm, you might have had to gasp for air, and you might even have even cried. These signs show just how much of a workout intense laughter can be. And, for most people, laughing really hard for twenty seconds is a lot more fun than rowing a boat for three minutes.

HUMOR IS A SKILL

Humor is a mind-set, a perspective, a way of looking at and thinking about situations and difficulties that allows a more relaxed and flexible approach to things. Humor triggers healing laughter. When under stress, however, or when not feeling well—and especially when suffering from serious illness—we tend to become sullen, rigid, pessimistic, and, well, humorless. The ability to laugh, like an unused muscle, can atrophy.

Fortunately, laughter can be restored. We needn't wait passively for humor to strike us. No matter how bad things are, we can still laugh. In fact, the worse things are, the more important it is that we laugh. Maintaining a humorous perspective is a skill that can be actively encouraged, cultivated, and practiced. It can be exercised and strengthened, like a muscle.

THE LAUGHING CLUB

A colorful example of intentionally exercising and sustaining the skill of laughter for health can be found in the renowned "Laughing Club of Calcutta," a group of men in India who regularly meet to perform physical exercises designed to stimulate laughter. They take long walks together on the beaches and through the streets, laughing all the way, and spreading the contagion of laughter. This ritual, based in the belief that laughter aids digestion, promotes health, and extends life, reflects an understanding of laughter's social nature as well as the notion that it can be developed intentionally. The speculation that at least some of these gentlemen assist their efforts with cannabis—the use of which is widespread at several levels of Indian society—remains unconfirmed.

FEAR OF SEEMING FOOLISH

Back on this side of the globe, the skills of laughter are practiced and taught by C. W. Metcalf and Roma Felible, authors of *Lighten Up: Survival Skills for People Under Pressure*. Metcalf and Felible identify the fear of appearing foolish as the predominant force that stifles humor, causing us to become "terminally serious"—constricted and uptight. Most people don't want to appear foolish or silly, and especially dread being witnessed in the process of being humiliated, fearing consequent loss of social credibility and status. For some people this fear is so extreme that it serves as the basis of a condition psychologists call "social phobia"—exaggerated, irrational fear of being embarrassed in front of others.

Metcalf and Felible's identification of fear of foolishness as laughter's prime enemy is supported by the research of University of Western Ontario psychologist Dr. Rod Martin. In his research into stress and humor, Martin found that adults laugh about seventeen times a day, whereas young children, who don't suffer from the fear of appearing foolish, laugh about three hundred times a day. To restore this high level of laughter and reap its healing benefits, we must overcome the fear of foolishness and act in the unselfconscious manner of small children playing childhood games.

WAYS OF ENCOURAGING LAUGHTER

"Childhood games" is a perfect description of the techniques that Metcalf and Felible offer for honing your humor skills and encouraging laughter. Like the Laughing Club of Calcutta, Metcalf and Felible employ specific physical exercises for making people laugh. Metcalf and Felible's methods are quick, easy, effective—and lots of fun. For the same reasons that the Laughing Club performs its rituals of humor collectively, these methods are best performed with a partner or in a group— your own private Laughing Club. Through the use of such exercises, you can learn to laugh *on purpose*.

The power of the laugh practice, of course, can be amplified by the laughter-promoting properties of cannabis, which help overcome social rigidity and restore a childlike immediacy of sensation that brings absurdity to the fore.

SMILE ON PURPOSE

When you smile you send a message to your emotional brain that something funny must be going on. Smiling "primes the pump" of good humor. The simple act of smiling generates positive feelings.

Metcalf and Felible suggest the following "smile exercise." Select a chair that you can stand up from quickly without losing your balance. Sit on the edge of the chair in a comfortable position. Count to three and, taking a deep breath, quickly stand up and smile as broadly as you can. Make sure that your teeth show. Sit back down and repeat the exercise several times. Soon, you will find yourself laughing. The bizarre, seemingly absurd nature of this exercise is part of its power to incite laughter.

MAKE FUNNY FACES

Stand or sit in front of a large mirror. Mirrored closet doors and full-length mirrors work well. Make faces at yourself in the mirror—the kinds of faces you would make to get a baby to laugh. Stick your tongue out and wag it. Make squealing and snorting noises. Use your hands to pull your cheeks out and push your nose up.

WATCH FUNNY MOVIES

As simple as it seems, according to Cousins this technique was crucial to his recovery from cancer. Watching funny movies is, of course, a particularly appropriate form of relief for periods of illness so intense as to render a person bedridden or incapable of going out or performing a great deal of activity. Watching films with people with similar taste in comedy will amplify their ability to elicit laughter. Alternatively, appropriate videotapes can also be left running in the background as you go about your daily activities; those moments when you stop to tune in to the action and dialogue or when the video grabs your attention may markedly increase the amount of humor and laughter that fills your day in a casual, unobtrusive way.

The promotion of humor and laughter and a distanced, light-hearted perspective on problems has long been a key motive for the use of cannabis. This aspect of the plant's psychoactivity is also part of its medicinal or healing value. While we've long understood the soothing effect of laughter on the psyche, science has only recently begun to show us how laughter also soothes and heals the body as well—providing us with further understanding of cannabis' healing magic.

CHAPTER 6

FAITH, HOPE, AND CANNABIS

*F*aith is an expectation that what we long for will come to be. Faith transcends belief. Whereas belief is a cognitive phenomenon, faith is spiritual, transcending fact, reason, and logic. Faith is trust in the mysterious power of the divine—whether Goddess or goddesses, God or gods, or higher self—to intervene and bring the miraculous or magical to fruition. Faith is the unexplainable but unmistakable *feeling* of closeness to or contact with a beneficent, divine force, the visceral trust that such an energy, spirit, or being is present, alive, potent, and active in human affairs.

Soren Kierkegaard, the nineteenth century Danish theologian considered to have been the first Existentialist philsosopher, defines despair as the "sickness unto death," in which the soul dies even though the body may remain alive. The only cure for despair, according to Kierkegaard, is a leap of faith, a leap beyond reason, and intellectual understanding to non-rational trust in the divine. It is through such faith, Kierkegaard maintains, that the soul finds eternal life. Faith is the personal relationship that connects the self to God—or what some of us today might prefer to call the higher self—whereas despair arises from severing the connection of faith. Faith alone, Kierkegaard says, restores the divine to the life of the individual, rekindling hope and dissolving despair.

Faith—in ourselves, our values and ideals, in God or some other transcendent force—makes it possible to truly *live* rather than merely to exist. Faith gives a sense of direction to the journey through life, and can quell fear of death. Without faith, as Kierkegaard emphasized, we are incomplete, disconcerted, adrift in a spiritual void.

Even the body benefits from faith. Faith fosters health and healing from disease. Cannabis—in its role as an *entheogen*, a substance with the capacity to generate inner experience of god or divinity—can assist in the restoration of faith and promote health. This is yet another aspect of the healing magic of cannabis.

FAITH PROMOTES HEALTH

Every civilization throughout history has had its form of faith. Today, according to a Gallup poll conducted in 1990, ninty-five percent of Americans profess belief in God, while seventy-six percent claim to pray regularly, fourteen percent of those polled in a telephone survey of 500 adults in Virginia believe that their bodies have been healed through prayer or divine intercession.

The feelings of well-being brought about by faith make an extraordinary contribution to health. Furthermore, religious and spiritual lifestyles are generally very healthy. As Herbert Benson, M.D., put it, "faith heals and makes the body whole. "

ANCIENT WISDOM

Throughout history, religious people and their leaders have offered testimony that faith has the power to heal. In the *New Testament* miraculous healings are attributed to the faith of the person healed rather than the powers of the putative healer. In the Gospel of Saint Luke, for example, Jesus says "Thy faith has made thee whole" to a woman who was healed of twelve years of bleeding upon touching his cloak, and he dismisses the thanks of a healed leper with exactly the same words. The implication is clear that Jesus located the responsibility for healing not in himself, but in the faith of those who had become whole. A priest who studied the many faith healings that have taken place at Lourdes, the famous Roman Catholic shrine in France, concluded that it is not miracles that produce faith, but rather faith that produces miracles.

Before recognizing a saint, the Catholic Church requires that doctors certify the validity of the healing miracles associated with the candidate for sainthood. In *Spontaneous Healing*, Weil, M.D., describes many of the miracles documented by the Church in the process of canonizing its saints. This documentation is an excellent source of information about the triggering of healing by faith. For example, Weil tells of a young man whose pathology report showed his body was riddled with cancer. After a visit to Lourdes, a second pathology report showed that he had *no cancer cells in his body*. His healing, attributed to faith, was totally unexplainable from a scientific perspective.

SCIENCE LOOKS AT FAITH

The connection between faith and health has been documented statistically. In *The Faith Factor,* a comprehensive review of scientific literature on the medical impact of spiritual experience, David Larson, M.D., shows correlations between religious factors and increased survival, lower blood pressure, reduced use of alcohol, cigarettes and other toxic drugs; reduced anger, anxiety, and depression, as well as better quality of life among those with cancer and heart disease. In a survey Larson found that cigarette smokers who regularly attended church—one indicator of faith—were four time less likely to have high blood pressure than smokers who did not attend church regularly. In fact, the average blood pressure of churchgoing smokers turned out to be about the same as that of non-smokers who didn't go to church. Larson also found that people who are religious report greater feelings of well-being, self-esteem, and altruism, as well as more satisfaction in marriage and life in general, than people who aren't religious.

Jeffrey Levin, M.D., of Eastern Virginia Medical School reviewed hundreds of epidemiological studies to conclude that faith in God lowers death rates and increases health. Thomas Oxman, M.D., and his colleagues at Dartmouth Medical School reported that among heart disease patients over the age of fifty-five who had open-heart surgery for either coronary artery or aortic valve disease, those who had spiritual faith were three times more likely to survive than those who did not.

The act of prayer both demonstrates faith and elicits feelings of faith. In a longitudinal study into the healing properties of prayer with sixty patients at the Arthritis Treatment Center, Dale Matthews, M.D., of the Georgetown University School of Medicine found remarkable improvement. For example. one patient who began the study with chronic pain throughout his body had no pain at all after six months, and no further need for medication.

Benson's research points to the health-enhancing properties of faith. Many of his patients reported spiritual feelings upon relaxing and as they continued to practice relaxation over time, the magnitude and intensity of these spiritual feelings tended to grow. Those who experienced feelings of faith showed remarkably greater medical benefits from practicing relaxation techniques than those who did not report spiritual feelings. As Benson put it, "a belief in God dispatched by our brains is deeply soothing to our bodies."

From faith emanates hope. Seligman's research demonstrated that hope is correlated with survival. Hope triggers the life force, summoning potentially Herculean strength into the struggle for survival. By serving as the wellspring of hope—especially the sort of non-rational, inexplicable hope that persists against all odds and flies against the logic of evidence—faith activates and strengthens the will to live. Hope promotes optimism and belief in positive possibilities, including the possibility of miraculous healing.

SCIENTIFIC RIGOR UNDERMINES FAITH

The scientific method is based on skepticism and doubt. In order for the result of a scientific study to be considered valid, for example, the null hypothesis must first be disproved. The null hypothesis is something like the "presumption of innocence" in court, by which the accused is presumed innocent until proven guilty beyond reasonable doubt. Similarly, the null hypothesis presumes that the result of an experiment is not meaningful until it is has been proven that it could not be a random occurrence.

In studies investigating medical treatments, the null hypothesis requires that the rate of improvement observed among patients be statistically significant—that is, sufficiently greater than what could occur by chance—if the benefit is to be attributed to the treatment. Additionally, to be taken seriously, a result must be reliably reproducible. However, even if a result *is* statistically significant *and* reproducible, it can still be dismissed as invalid if *any* flaw, no matter how small, can be found in the design of the experiment.

MIRACLES HAPPEN

There are, however, unproven treatments that *do* work—and *continue* to work whether or not they've passed the scrutiny of science. Similarly, "miraculous" recoveries continue to take place against all odds. Science, however, is blind to their wonders. Because their occurrence is rare, they are dismissed as random events. And because miracles don't occur on command, they can't be reproduced. For these reasons, miracles don't appear in the picture of the world drawn by science. Nonetheless, miracles do happen—and are no less miraculous for occurring outside the methodological boundaries of scientific experimentation.

SKEPTICISM

Because of the absence of the miraculous in the scientific worldview, the value placed on scientific outlook in our culture makes it easy to lose faith. Science has assumed such a god-like position that the skepticism and doubt built into the scientific method—the presumption of the null hypothesis—have become ingrained in our educational system, in the forms of critical analysis taught in our schools, and in the way we view life. In short, our culture has developed a negative mind-set that makes it increasingly difficult to have faith—in anything.

DOCTORS WITHOUT FAITH

This skepticism is integral to the education received by doctors. The frightening result is that the health practitioners in whom we place *our* faith and trust have been brainwashed into faithlessness. Doctors unwittingly communicate, in the manner of a contagion, a lack of faith in the possibility of extraordinary, miraculous recovery and healing.

The hopelessness so communicated to their patients, as Seligman's work shows, is not only deleterious to health, but can engender a despair that wields lethal power.

The ubiquitous absence of faith within the milieu of medical practice does not bode well for health, and negatively influences chances of recovery from illness. More than ever before, it becomes paramount to find ways of generating faith.

FAITH EMANATES FROM THE QUIET MIND

To experience faith, we must first quiet the activity of the linear, rational, verbal domain of the psyche, called the rational mind, that dominates awareness during waking hours. The rational mind thinks in words and generates an ongoing internal conversation so constant that we are often unaware of it. This internal mental noise, much of it a product of familial, social, and cultural conditioning, continually reindoctrinates with beliefs, often very negative ones, that may not have been examined in years and may no longer hold true. Teachers of Eastern meditative techniques sometimes refer to this compulsive mentation as the incessant chatter of the "monkey mind."

The monkey mind's ceaseless activity blocks the nonrational, intuitive aspect of the psyche from which the experience of faith comes. Stilling the monkey mind, therefore, helps us to contact the "quiet mind," alternatively called the higher self, the inner wellspring of wisdom and strength that gives rise to feelings of faith, sensations of contact with spiritual energy, and closeness to God.

QUIETING THE MONKEY MIND

Discontinuing the mental activity we normally call "thought," however, is not so easy! If you like, just try it for a moment. Put down this book and simply stop thinking. Stop words and thoughts from happening in your mind—just for a few moments. Go ahead!

Not so easy, eh? Fortunately there's a trick that can be used to silence the stream of words babbling through the rational mind. The rational mind is linear, not simultaneous, in the way that it functions. It can think only in one set of words at a time. Multiple sets of words can't appear in the mind in the same moment. Therefore, feeding the mind a chosen word or phrase, focusing upon it, and repeating it over and over, either silently or aloud, will short-circuit mental chatter, stilling the monkey mind.

This simple but powerful method is at the root of contemplative techniques like mantra meditation, in which a phrase with spiritual meaning is repeated over and over in the mind, repetitive chants such as those performed by Hindus and Christian monks, and many forms of prayer. It is also the principle behind the standard techniques taught by Benson and others for eliciting relaxation. Other techniques used involve repetitive, rhythmic body motions that provide the mind with a center of focus, such as rocking back and forth and shifting the weight of the body from one foot to the other; or to the graceful, fluid, circular motions of "soft form" martial arts such as Tai Chi, for example.

CANNABIS CAN HELP GENERATE FAITH

Cannabis is an entheogen. This term, popularized largely through the efforts of ethnobotanical researcher Dr. Jonathan Ott, means literally "generating god within" and refers to substances that can facilitate religious experiences and feelings of spirituality. Stronger psychedelics like peyote, mescaline, psilocybin, and LSD are also entheogens.

The psychoactivity of cannabis can assist in quieting the mind to contact the inner source of faith and hope. Cannabis aids in eliciting the relaxation integral to spiritual, meditative, and contemplative techniques, and its mental effects are associated with the intuitive, imagistic, nonrational, nonlinear aspect of the psyche from which flow faith and hope.

The tradition of using cannabis as an entheogen stretches back thousands of years. In India, cannabis is associated with the Hindu god Shiva. Bhang, a drink made from cannabis, is considered "the heavenly guide" and "the food of the gods" by certain Hindu sects who have long used the plant as an adjunct to meditation and the study of scripture. Yogis recount using bhang to "center their thoughts on the eternal" and many Hindu saints used cannabis for "fixing the mind on god." Fakirs and ascetics, India's wandering practitioners of extreme religious austerity, used cannabis to facilitate communication with their deities. The Japanese traditionally burned cannabis in marriage ceremonies to drive away evil spirits, and members of the mystical Sufi sect of Islam used cannabis for spiritual insight.

CATALYST OF THE NEW AGE MOVEMENT

Cannabis' entheogenic properties played a significant role in the explosion of the plant's use in the 1960s. A crucial early event was the "Good Friday Experiment" conducted at Harvard by Dr. Timothy Leary and his colleagues, in which students of Divinity were administered LSD in a religious setting to produce "trips" whose characteristics closely resembled those of classic religious and mystical experiences. As the decade unfolded, such spiritually-charged LSD experiences helped catalyze widespread interest in alternative and Eastern religious and spiritual forms such as Zen Buddhism and Taoism, and fueled fascination with Indian masters of yoga among western followers.

These developments, taking root in the counterculture and blossoming in later decades as the New Age movement, were crucially supported by the entheogenic qualities of cannabis. The plant offered a relatively brief and non-threatening initiation into psychoactivity. Where LSD was generally considered appropriate only for occasional use, cannabis could be used more regularly to recall the spiritual intensity of LSD experiences and help nurture, maintain, and integrate into daily life the insights they yielded. Cannabis is often used with the religious rituals, ceremonies, and meditative forms widely explored as alternative spiritualities proliferated, and in this capacity played a formative role in awakening spiritual inclinations among many who never used LSD. Stephen Gaskin, a major American proponent of alternative spirituality and founder of the long-lived Tennessee countercultural commune called "The Farm", discusses the continuing contemporary entheogenic use of cannabis in his book, *Cannabis Spirituality*.

Two Seekers Who Got High

Two Seekers enjoyed meeting after dinner to smoke cannabis and discuss their progress in seeking the quiet mind.

"Some people think that getting high is not spiritual," said the First Seeker. "I wonder how we can integrate getting high with seeking the quiet mind? I'll ask the Shaman."

So the First Seeker went to the Shaman. "Shaman Woman, I am devoted to seeking my quiet mind, but I like to get high with my friend as well. Would it be okay if I get high when I am seeking my quiet mind?" he asked.

Enraged, the Shaman waved the Seeker away, grumbling "All you care about is getting high! Get out of here!"

Shaken, the First Seeker scurried back to his friend. "Don't talk about getting high to the Shaman," he warned. "She's not into it!"

"Humm, I'll talk to her," said the Second Seeker. He went to see the Shaman.

"Shaman Woman, I am devoted to seeking my quiet mind and I enjoy getting high with my friend. Would it be okay for me to seek my quiet mind when I'm high?" asked the Second Seeker.

"Yes, you should always seek your quiet mind," the Shaman Woman said, nodding approvingly, "especially when you're high!"

Simply "smoking dope" doesn't automatically awaken feelings of faith or inspire experiences of God. On the other hand, cannabis, used in a meditative setting with commitment and discipline, can amplify the techniques used to reach the quiet mind and awaken the faith that calls forth miracles.

CANNABIS AND VISUALIZATION TECHNIQUES

Oncologists Carl O. Simonton, M.D., and Stephanie Simonton have shown that using intuitively-based imagery, like that of a video-game "pacman" eating cancer cells, or of a white knight slaying black dragons of cancer, is useful in fighting the disease. The psychoactivity of cannabis facilitates working with the intuitive, imagistic, nonlogical processes that are the basis of such visualizations or autogenic healing techniques.

Cannabis makes it easier to slow down, relax, and to visualize images vividly, and in detail. Having faith in the effectivenss of such techniques comes a littler easier when using cannabis, increasing the likelihood that a person will practice them regularly while it sends a non-verbal message of positive belief to the cells and organs of the body that helps empower the techniques themselves.

USING CANNABIS WITH PRAYER

Repetition of a word or phrase, silently or aloud, stills the chatter of the mind, relaxing the body and quieting the mind. Often spiritual feelings come to the fore. This technique is integral to the practice of prayer. Interestingly, Benson found that most people chose words of religious or spiritual meaning with which to practice relaxation. Fur-thermore, many of his patients reported spiritual feelings when they achieved a relaxed state, whether or not they used words of spiritual import.

HOW PRAYER WORKS

Using words of spiritual meaning increases the faith-arousing power of techniques for reaching into the quiet mind, and is the essence of prayer. The combination of stilling the monkey mind to bring forth the quiet mind, while simultaneously evoking faith with the words used, helps explain how prayer works.

As many of the yogis, worshipers of Shiva, and spiritual pilgrims of India have long known, the entheogenic properties of cannabis can further enhance the power of prayer to arouse faith. The power of prayer can be amplified even more by composing and using a prayer that is of special, personal meaning, one that uses words that have particular relevance one's situation and special faith-evoking power for the individual. Such a prayer can be composed by beginning with a favorite traditional prayer and tailoring the phrases and passages to have special personal significance and meaning. This technique enhances the prayer's potency for the person. In addition to using cannabis as an adjunct to the act of prayer, cannabis can be useful for facilitating inspiration in the process of composing the prayer itself.

A friend created a personal prayer to Saint Sebastian, whose strength of faith he admired. He started with the traditional Christian prayer to Saint Joseph he had learned as a child and which was especially meaningful to him. Here is the original prayer to Saint Joseph.

Prayer to Saint Joseph

O Saint Joseph, whose protection is so great, so strong, so prompt before the throne of God, I place in you all my interest and desires. O Saint Joseph, do assist me by your powerful intercession, and obtain for me from your Divine Son all spiritual blessings, through Jesus Christ, our Lord. So that, having engaged here below your heavenly power, I may offer my thanksgiving and homage to the most loving of Fathers. O Saint Joseph, I never grow tired of contemplating you, and Jesus asleep in your arms; I dare not approach while He reposes near your heart. Press him in my name and kiss His dear head for me and ask Him to return the kiss when I draw my dying breath. Amen. O Saint Joseph, hear my prayers and obtain my petitions. O Saint Joseph, pray for me.

Regina Press
Reproduction: 35-1501

The prayer's personal meaning comes from Sebastian's given name, Joseph, which was taken from Saint Joseph, the stepfather to Jesus, and he has an important stepfather-type relationship. As a teenager, he began calling himself Sebastian, which evolved into the name everyone who knows him uses.

Saint Sebastian was a Roman centurian who had secretly con-verted to Christianity. He healed many people, including the mayor of Rome, who then similarly converted to Christianity. Emporer Diocletian was enraged by this and ordered this soldiers to kill Sebastian. They tied him to a tree, shot him full of arrows and left him for dead. But Saint Sebastian's faith was so great that he did not die. Here is Sebastian's personal prayer to Saint Sebastian, adapted from the prayer to Saint Joseph.

Prayer to Saint Sebastian

O Saint Sebastian, I pray for the courage of your spirit.
Shot full of arrows you survive death through the strength
of faith. O valiant Roman centurion, turned Christian
pacifist, lend me your blessing of faith to survive my healing
crisis and find the path of wellness. Amen.

The prayer asks that Saint Sebastian will bestow his strength of faith which the petitioner needs in his stuggle to overcome cancer and return to wellness.

In composing a personal prayer, you might choose to pray to a deity, saint, or archetypal figure that embodies the quality you desire. For instance, you might pray to a lion for strength and courage, to an eagle for breadth and clarity of vision, to the Goddess Quan Yin for compassion, or to a mountain for endurance.

Alternatively, you could use the Twenty-Third Psalm of David as a starting point. Its powerful, familiar images tend to evoke feelings of faith, even among many who have no affinity with the Judeo-Christian religious tradition in which it originates.

For another prayer, we return to the theme of the inspiring faith with entheogenic substances. While in India in 1965, Dr. Timothy Leary, using the entheogenic qualities of LSD and cannabis was inspired by the

Chinese spiritual text, the *Tao Te Ching*. to write *Psychedelic Prayers*. One of those prayers deals with the quiet mind and awakening of faith and hope.

He Who Knows The Center Endures

Who knows the outside is clever
Who knows the center endures
Who masters others gains robot power
Who comes to the center has flowering strength

Faith of consciousness is freedom
Hope of consciousness is strength
Love of consciousness evokes the same in return

Faith of seed frees
Hope of seed flowers
Love of seed grows

ILLNESS AS A TRANSFORMATIVE OPPORTUNITY

Spiritual understanding of disease held by shamans, sages, and healers throughout time has reflected the concept of illness as a healing opportunity. The phrase "healing crisis," used instead of the word "disease," reflects this point of view. Here illness is seen as an opportunity to undertake a journey that penetrates the underworld of causes of disease and suffering in a person's life and, on the archetypal level, the causes of human suffering and disease altogether. Through this healing journey these causes are confronted and overcome with the help of spiritual guides, allies, and the person's access to universal healing life force.

The person emerges from the "disease" into a higher state of wellness, a deeper understanding of life, and greater personal capacities than before. The classic journey of shamanic initiation describes the healing crisis through which members of traditional tribal cultures must pass in order to become healers and practitioners of native medicinal arts. Incidentally, the shaman's healing arts often involve the use of psychoactive plants.

Understanding disease as an opportunity for personal growth—expressed in the homily "every pain and suffering is a blessing in disguise"—is embodied in the ancient Chinese spiritual manual on the conduct of life, the *I Ching*, also called *Book of Changes*, in which the symbol for "crisis" is the same as the symbol for "opportunity." The writings collected in the *I Ching* emerge in large part from the Taoist tradition of Chinese culture, known for its sophisticated practice of healing arts including the use of herbs to activate the body's latent healing energy or *Chi*. (Incidentally, the Taoist tradition employed cannabis as a medicine). The Taoist practitioner of healing arts is a wise man described as a magician and spiritual teacher.

Faith is key to weathering the healing crisis to achieve personal transformation. From faith comes the strength to face the pain and fear presented by illness. Illness can test, temper, and build faith, spurring spiritual transformation. Faith itself may be the factor that makes it possible for personal transformation to emerge from the maelstrom of disease, for faith calls forth miracles, and personal transformation can be miraculous.

People threatened with illness are sometimes reluctant to call upon faith to heal them or even to soothe them, as if to do so would somehow compromise a realistic grasp of their situations. But having faith does not mean relinquishing common sense or informed decision-making. And having faith does not require forgoing conventional medical treatment. Faith is not an escape from reality, but a means of shaping reality, present and future, and an important resource for healing. There is nothing to lose in calling upon faith. It can only help.

ENTHEOGENIC USE OF CANNABIS

If the use of a plant can facilitate faith, it can facilitate healing. In light of its long history of entheogenic use and the testimonies of thousands who have employed it in this capacity, cannabis is clearly such a plant. The inspiration of feelings of faith and contact with spiritual energies is central to cannabis' healing magic. Cannabis can be used in conjunction with prayer, meditation, visualization, and other spiritual practices to heighten and amplify their efficacy. Its use can help engender sensations of quietude, awe, wonder at the beauty of nature, internal illumination, and connectedness with the cosmos.

PART TWO

CHAPTER 7

PREPARING CANNABIS

There are three basic methods for making medicinal use of the active ingredients in the cannabis plant: inhalation, oral ingestion, and topical application. To better understand the advantages and disadvantages of each of these methods, and whether a given method may be more or less appropriate depending on circumstances, it is helpful to know which parts of the plant contain the highest concentrations of active ingredients and to know how these active ingredients—called *cannabinoids*—are absorbed by the body. No matter which of these methods of administering cannabis is chosen, the same initial procedures for preparing and storing it will help in making the most efficient medicinal use of the plant.

HOW CANNABIS' INGREDIENTS ARE ABSORBED

Microscopic hair-like stalks found on the surfaces of the leaves, stems, and flowers of the cannabis plant produce a resin that contains cannabinoids. These stalks, which are not found on the roots or seeds of the plant, are most highly concentrated on the *bracts*, small sheaths which surround and protect the embryonic seeds of the female flower. So, while it is possible to use leaves and stems for smoking, it is preferable to use the flowers because smaller amounts of this part of the plant can be smoked to deliver the same quantity of active ingredients that would require greater amounts of leaf or stem. Additionally, while the smoke from leaves is usually quite smooth and palatable, the smoke from stems is harsh and irritating. Leaves and stems, however, are valuable in making preparations for oral ingestion, where minimizing the amount of plant matter used is not a health issue as it is with smoking preparations.

Most cannabanoids, including THC, are not water-soluble. In order to be absorbed into the body, therefore, these cannabinoids must first either be vaporized as in smoking, or extracted by agents that dissolve oils, such as fats, alcohols, or other oils.

Our bodies expend considerably more metabolic effort assimilating cannabinoid-carrying fats and oils than cannabinoids which have been vaporized. Consequently, it takes much longer for cannabinoids to be absorbed by eating than by smoking. The variabilities involved in the process of absorbing cannabinoid-containing fats or oils, and the length of time required before the full effects of such absorption are felt, make it difficult to determine a standard dose for oral ingestion. Cannabinoids are more rapidly, efficiently, and predictably absorbed through inhalation, making it easier to control one's dosage. Smoking, however, presents health concerns that must be taken into consideration.

Cannabinoids can also be absorbed through the skin into localized areas of the body when plant matter is applied directly to the skin in the form of a salve or poultice. This method is known as topical application, and has limited use for certain conditions such as arthritis, dermatitis, or skin infections. Since cannabinoids are absorbed through topical application only into the areas of the body where applied, they are not delivered to the central nervous system. This method, therefore, does not result in a psychoactive experience.

PREPARING CANNABIS FOR MEDICAL USE

Instructions for preparation and use are provided for those using cannabis as a healing aid in districts where medical use of marijuana is sanctioned. It is also provided for doctors and other health practioniers and any other persons needing use information, as provided by the First Amendement of the U.S. Constitution. The authors and the publisher caution readers against breaking the law, including unlawful or "recreational" use of cannabis. An excellent resource is *Marijuana Law* by Richard Glen Boire.

Medical quality cannabis comes in the form of small, dried flower buds which are usually seedless which is called "sinsemillia" or without seeds. Preparation begins with the removal of the small leaves and flowers from the stem. The flowers are removed from the stem by crumbling with the fingers, or they may be cut from the stem with a pair of fine scissors. Any large leaves on the flowers may be smoked, but since they are less potent than the flowers, it may be preferable to set them aside for use in food preparations such as cannabis butter. Large stems can be discarded, but relatively small ones can also be used in cannabis butter.

REMOVING SEEDS AND STEMS

Lesser grades of cannabis have a higher percentage of leaves with a lot of seeds and stems. The seeds and stems can be removed by crumbling the cannabis in a tray, then tilting it up at about a 20° angle, gently tapping or shaking the tray so that the seeds roll down to the bottom. Remaining seeds can be separated by raking the powdered cannabis upward with an open matchbook or credit cArd so the seeds roll down.

Another way of removing seeds and stems is to sift the mixture through a fine metal screen, such as a tea strainer and other kitchen sieve. The weave of the screen should be large enough to allow small bits of crushed plant matter, but not so larage as to allow seeds to pass through. Pressing the mixture gently against the screen with the fingers in a circular motion grinds the plant matter into powder small enough to pass through the screen. When all the seeds and stems are removed, the cannabis is ready to use.

STORING CANNABIS

Exposure to light, heat, and air contribute to the deterioration of the active ingredients in cannabis. Therefore, cannabis is best stored in an airtight container like a Mason jar or film canister and kept in a dark place at room temperature.

To know how to best utilize cannabis for a particular condition in a particular individual, whether one might best smoke, eat or apply cannabis to the skin—depends upon knowing how the medicinial ingredients are distributed in the plant and how they are differentially absorbed depending upon the method of use. By performing a few simple steps, cannabis can be prepared and stored to maximize its medicinial usefullness.

CHAPTER 8

INHALATION METHODS

The effects of cannabis are felt fastest when it is inhaled. Cannabis can be inhaled by smoking it in a cigarette, pipe, or waterpipe, or by using a vaporizer. Each inhalation method has advantages and disadvantages.

PROS AND CONS OF SMOKING

Inhalation by smoking is the most common way to use cannabis with the advantages of quick action, convenience, ease of monitoring the amount ingested, the small chance of accidentally ingesting too much, and short term duration of effects. Inhalation is especially appropriate for those suffering from severe nausea or loss of appetite, who may have difficulty eating or keeping medicines down long enough for them to take effect.

The idea of smoking cannabis and all the health issues that entails defeats the purpose for many people of using this safe, natural plant remedy. Some may be concerned about increased risk of bronchitis. Worse, long-term smoking of cannabis may be a precipitating factor in mouth and throat cancer. People with asthma, chronic bronchitis, shortness of breath, allergy or other negative reaction to smoke, or who are just personally averse to smoking, all have reason to avoid this common method of administering cannabis as medicine. Nonetheless, smoking is appropriate in severe nausea or loss of appetite.

Cannabis smoke may also be irritating to others, especially non-smokers. Additionally, the powerful and distinctive odor of burning cannabis risks detection by law enforcement officers.

If you choose smoking it is smart to inhale as little smoke as necessary to obtain the desired effects which means using the most potent cannabis available, such as high-grade sensimilla flower buds or hashish.

Contrary to popular belief, there's no reason to hold a "hit" (or inhalation) of cannabis smoke in the lungs as long as possible to get the most from it. Cannabinoids from the smoke pass almost instantly into the body through the lungs. Holding the smoke in the lungs any longer than a few seconds increases the lung's exposure to irritants.

CANNABIS CIGARETTES

The main advantage of hand-rolled cannabis cigarettes, called "joints", is convenience. They are easy to carry around and easy to consume. The papers in which the cigarettes are rolled, however, burn at a higher temperature than the cannabis itself, resulting in a hotter smoke that may increase irritation to the throat and respiratory system. Tests show that smoking cannabis in cigarettes is a somewhat less efficient means of delivering cannabinoids than smoking cannabis in a pipe. Additionally, rolling papers often contain harmful chemical additives included to bleach the paper and control burning.

ROLLING A CANNABIS CIGARETTE

Rolling papers used to make cigarettes come in a surprising variety and are readily available in liquor stores, head shops and cannabis buyers clubs. When you pull out a paper you'll notice that it has a gummed edge and a lengthwise crease down the middle. To roll a cigarette a rolling paper is opened up flat, with the crease running left to right and the gummed surface on the far edge. A second, parallel fold is created in the bottom half of the paper by folding it so that the edge is even with the crease in the middle. When the rolling paper is opened back up, the two folds create a curved effect in the paper, ready to cradle the powdered cannabis, which is sprinkled along the crease closest to the paper's bottom edge and distributed evenly along the crease except at the ends, where leaving a tiny empty margin will help prevent cannabis from falling out when the cigarette is rolled. The short flap of the rolling paper (the part between second crease and the bottom edge) is folded over the cannabis, and then gently but firmly rolled back and forth, with the thumbs and forefingers of both hands, between the two folds. During this phase of rolling a cigarette, the upper half of the paper (with the gummed edge along the top) is kept free. The up-and-down rolling begins with the thumbs touching at the center of the cigarette but brings them further apart with each rolling motion until the cigarette is held with the thumbs apart at the ends. This rolling action slowly packs the cannabis into a long, thin, even tube-like shape.

Sometimes cannabis spills out the ends of the cigarette. In this case, the cigarette is slowly unrolled so that the cannabis can be gently pushed back towards the center of the cigarette. Rolling of the cigarette is then resumed, beginning with thumbs touching in the center and then moving outward. When thumbs get to the edge of the cigarette, the gummed strip is licked and the cigarette is rolled all the way up to the top edge, using all of the paper. Gently rubbing the dry side of the gummed edge will seal the cigarette, which after a moment's drying is ready to smoke.

Rolling Is An Art

Rolling a good joint is an art. If the cigarette is too tightly packed, it will be hard to draw smoke through and it will stop burning. If rolled too loosely, it will burn unevenly and fall apart. One trick is using wired rolling papers which are purchased in buyer's clubs and smoke shops. Wired papers have a thin wire glued along the non-gummed edge. The stiffness of the wire makes rolling the cigarette easier. The wire facilitates airflow along the length of the cigarette, helping it to burn more evenly and avoiding "runs"—burns that run up the length of the cigarette along one side. Finally, the wire acts as a handle so that the joint can be smoked to the very end without burning fingers.

A cigarette rolling machine is a small, inexpensive apparatus that can be purchased at most smoke shops and some cannabis buyer's clubs. This device, which comes with instructions, can be used for quick and neat rolling of evenly-packed, easily-smoked cannabis cigarettes. Most rolling machines are designed for tobacco cigarettes which require considerably more plant material. Using a cigarette machine with cannabis yields a beautiful cigarette that is expensive and wasteful since it takes only a few inhalations or "drags" of good medicinal sinsemellia to obtain beneficial effects.

PIPES

Like tobacco, cannabis can also be smoked in pipes. Cannabis pipes, however have smaller bowls than tobacco pipes. Some cannabis pipes have small metal lids that screw onto the bowl, keeping the cannabis and ash confined within and preventing ash and bits of cannabis from falling out into purses, backpacks, pockets, etc. Sometimes lids have small holes that allow smoking with the lid on, minimizing the escape of odorous smoke.

PROS AND CONS OF PIPES

Using a pipe to smoke cannabis avoids the inhalation of chemicals present in rolling papers, and allows lower burning temperatures with the result of a cooler smoke that is less irritating to the throat and respiratory system. Smoking a pipe also makes more efficient use of the active ingredients in cannabis, allowing a higher percentage to be delivered into the body than with cannabis cigarettes.

On the other hand, pipes may be more difficult than cigarettes to dispose of quickly and easily should it be necessary to do so. Furthermore, pipes can be easily analyzed for cannabis residues in law enforcement laboratories, be considered "paraphernalia," and serve as evidence of unlawful use of cannabis. For a detailed discussion of this issue see *Marijuana Law* by attorney Richard Glen Boire.

HOW PIPES ARE USED

Cannabis pipes can be purchased at hemp stores, smoke shops, and head shops which specialize in the retailing of materials related to the recreational use of cannabis.

A pinch of finely crumbled or cut cannabis can be placed in the bowl and lit immediately. The most efficient and healthful way to smoke cannabis in a pipe is to load the bowl with a pinch of cannabis large enough only for one or two inhalations—thus minimizing the generation of ash—while taking care to light it gently from an indirect flame. The heat of a direct flame destroys many of the cannabinoids, which are best preserved for inhalation by holding the flame at the maximum distance that allows the herbal material to catch fire. Some people habitually re-ignite and smoke the ash for a few inhalations after it is already spent in an effort to get the most out of their expensive medicine. This practice is futile; cannabis ash contains inconsequentially minute quantities of cannabinoids, and much larger amounts of irritants.

CLEAN PIPES OFTEN

Cannabis pipes clog up quickly with tars and smoke waste. A dark brown, viscous residue with an unpleasant taste accumulates in the bowl. Pipes must, therefore, be cleaned often. A pipe that can be taken apart allows easier cleaning of the bowl. Alcohol will dissolve tars, and a paper towel can be used to wipe the bowl clean before reassembling it. Pipe cleaners dipped in alcohol can be used to clean the stem. Screens can be changed as often as they become saturated with residue.

Unlike tobacco pipes, cannabis pipes contain a fine-weave screen at the bottom of the bowl to prevent inhalation of ash and burning material. Extra screens, which can be purchased very inexpensively at the kinds of retail establishments mentioned, are kept on hand to replace screens that have developed holes or become clogged and saturated with ash and smoking resins.

WATERPIPES

The middle eastern "hookah" or waterpipe is a favorite way to smoke. Waterpipes are made of a spherical or cylindrical flask-like chamber that is filled a third to halfway with water. Atop the chamber is a pipe-type bowl for smoking, which holds a fine-mesh screen of the same kind as that used in a cannabis pipe. A tube or stem extends vertically from the bottom of the bowl down into the chamber, ending submerged in the water. The stem through which one draws the smoke goes into the side of the chamber, ending above the water level. Inhalation draws the smoke down from the bowl through the water where it bubbles up into the air chamber where it is drawn into the stems and inhaled.

"Bongs" are variations of the waterpipe with oversized, cylindrical, open-topped chambers designed to make possible the inhalation of huge amounts of smoke in a single draw taken directly into the mouth from the chamber. Because of the size of the inhalations, they are not generally considered appropriate for medicinal use of cannabis.

PROS AND CONS OF WATERPIPES

The advantage of waterpipes is that the smoke is cooled by being drawn through water. Hot smoke can sear off the tops of the *cilia*, tiny hair-like fibers that line respiratory passageways and direct and regulate mucus flow with their waving motion. Searing of the cilia by hot smoke can result in congestion.

There is some about the effectiveness of waterpipes in removing tars and irritants from smoke. Research sponsored by MAPS (Multidisciplinary Association for Psychedelic Studies) and California NORML (National Organization for Reform of Marijuana Laws), found that waterpipes filter out more active THC than irritating tars. Use of waterpipes therefore requires that more cannabis be smoked to achieve an effect that could be reached by smoking less cannabis in a pipe or cigarette. The result is exposure to greater amounts of smoke, and therefore greater amounts of smoke toxins, tending to cancel out health benefits that might be gained by filtering the smoke through water. Like pipes, according to law waterpipes can be considered evidence of illegal use of cannabis.

USING A WATERPIPE

The chamber is filled with enough water to cover the bottom of the stem or tube that descends into the chamber from the pipe bowl, but the surface of the water must remain sufficiently clear of the opening of the stem through which the smoke is inhaled to prevent inhalation from drawing water into it.

For smoking, the bowl is packed tightly with a small amount of cannabis. As with pipes, the flame is best held at the maximum distance that permits ignition. A long, slow, steady inhalation is best for igniting the cannabis and drawing it through the filtering water.

As with any pipe, a waterpipe should be cleaned regularly, including changing the water and replacing the screen. The waterpipe selected should be easily taken apart for cleaning. Pipe cleaners soaked in alcohol can be used to clean the tubes and stems, a paper towel and alcohol for cleaning the bowl, and the inside of the chamber can be soaked in alcohol, cleaned out with a wire brush, and rinsed with water.

VAPORIZERS

Vaporizers gently heat cannabis to a temperature at which the cannabinoid-containing resins become vaporized—but not so hot that they are incinerated, as is the case when a flame lights the cannabis in pipes, waterpipes, and cigarettes. Vaporization does not destroy the active ingredients in the plant. Furthermore, potentially carcinogenic particles, which are byproducts of incineration, are not released with the vapor because it hasn't been exposed to a flame.

Vaporizers consist of a large glass sphere containing a heating element on which the cannabis is placed. When the cannabis reaches the point of vaporization, the sphere fills with mist. A long plastic tube extruding from inside the glass sphere is used for inhaling the vaporized cannabinoids. Commercially manufactured vaporizers come with detailed instructed for the assembly, use, and maintenance of the device.

PROS AND CONS OF VAPORIZERS

The MAPS and California NORML research concluded that vaporizers are the most effective means of smoking cannabis. The vaporizer outscored all other smoking devices in removal of tars. An additional advantage of the vaporizer is that fumes remain entirely contained within the device, so that medicinal cannabinoids are not lost through dissipation into the surrounding air, and much less odor is generated than by cannabis cigarettes, pipes, and waterpipes.

There is some evidence that although vaporizers are a less efficient means of consuming THC which is the cannabinoid that causes the high, they do instead deliver a higher percentage of a therapeutic cannabinoid called CBN. Much of the THC loss may be due to oxidation occurring inside the vaporizer. Further studies are required to understand and perhaps correct this effect. By law, vaporizers, like pipes and waterpipes, can be considered evidence of illegal use of cannabis.

Each inhalation method has its own advantages and disadvantages in terms of health, legal issues, efficiency, and convenience. All smoking methods are fairly simple and straightforward, and can be easily learned. Which method is used is a matter of individual choice. None of these methods are exclusive of the others; different methods may be appropriate for different occasions and circumstances. Among those new to the various methods of medicinal use of cannabis, some patient experimentation will reveal which ones are easiest and most appropriate for a particular person.

CHAPTER 9

CANNABIS FOODS

Many individuals who do not want to smoke can nonetheless gain the important medical benefits of cannabis' healing magic. All of the therapeutic actions achieved by smoking are also available through eating cannabis in foods.

In fact, eating cannabis can be more effective than smoking it in relieving pain and reducing inflammation. The therapeutic action lasts longer when cannabis is eaten (up to twelve hours), an advantage in situations that don't allow smoking cannabis. Eating foods prepared from high-quality cannabis provides an extraordinarily soothing effect. For some patients eating cannabis offers a level and quality of relief that simply can't be achieved by smoking it.

DRAWBACKS OF EATING CANNABIS

Nevertheless, eating cannabis does have some drawbacks in comparison with smoking. When eaten, cannabis takes thirty to ninety minutes to take effect, as opposed to a few minutes when smoked, which means it's easier to accidentally ingest too much cannabis when it's eaten. When smoking one can make a puff-by-puff adjustment of intake as soon as the desired level of medicinal activity has been achieved. Another drawback is that if too much cannabis is eaten excessive effects will last longer than when too much is smoked. Another problem with eating is when too little cannabis is eaten, the ineffectiveness of the dose doesn't become apparent for an hour or more. And even if this situation is remedied by eating more cannabis, full therapeutic action won't kick in for perhaps *another* hour or more. For a person depending upon cannabis for relief of significant pain, such miscalculation and delay of relief can amount to more than mere inconvenience.

Fortunately, however, a brief period of experimentation with cooking and eating cannabis is usually all that's required. It doesn't take long to learn how much to include in a food recipe and how much of that food to eat in order to achieve optimal medicinal effects.

"BROWNIE" MARY RATHBUN

Mary Rathbun is a heroine of the medical marijuana movement, well known for her tireless efforts to provide cannabis brownies to sick people in the San Francisco area. She was the first volunteer on the AIDS ward at San Francisco General Hospital and baked "pot brownies" for the patients. Mary was arrested three times for this clandestine behavior. The media adoringly portrayed her as a cheerful, feisty grandma personality. Twice charges against her were dropped, partly due to the media's sympathetic coverage depicting a battle pitting this lovable grandma against heartless police depriving sick people of their beneficial cookies.

The San Francisco Board of Supervisors declared August 25, 1992 "Brownie Mary Day" in honor of her decade of volunteer work with AIDS patients. In collaboration with Dennis Peron, founder of the San Francisco Cannabis Buyer's Club, she coauthored *Brownie Mary's Marijuana Cookbook / Dennis Peron's Recipe for Social Change*, the book from which the table of dosages and the two Brownie Mary recipes were adapted.

DOSE PER PERSON ACCORDING TO BROWNIE MARY

Below is an adaptation of Brownie Mary's table of cannabis dosages for one person. Appetite stimulation, which is generally desired by AIDS patients and those undergoing cancer chemotherapy, is accompanied by a mild psychoactive high. A higher doses provides a more psychoactive type of experience, suited to the visualization and imagery work described in the relaxation and wellness exercises included in this book. Experienced medicinal users who have developed some skill in working with cannabis' effects often seek this dosage level; novice medicinal users may want to start out with smaller amounts.

	Appetite Stimulant	Psychedelic
Marijuana leaf	1/2 gram	2 grams
Imported marijuana flowers	1/4 gram	1 gram
Hashish*	1/8 gram	1 gram
Sinsemilla flowers	1/8 gram	2 grams

*Potency of hashish varies widely.
Recipes using hashish should be avoided by novice cooks.

EXTRACTING THC WITH BUTTER

THC and other active cannabinoids will dissolve in fats and oils such as those found in common household butter. In fact, cannabis butter, often called "cannabutter," is one of the most popular and widely used ways of extracting the active ingredients from cannabis for use in foods. It is usually made with leaf trimmed from freshly harvested buds. Leaves are less potent and therefore less suitable for smoking than the buds themselves, but are quite adequate for use in butter. Cannabutter can be added to any recipe calling for butter.

CANNABUTTER

Pulverize leaves in a blender or mortar. Melt approximately twice as much butter by weight as cannabis on low heat, taking care not to burn it. Slowly stir powdered cannabis leaf into melted butter. Simmer on low heat for approximately twelve hours.
As liquid in mix evaporates, add water a cup at a time to insure that water-soluble cannabinoids will also be extracted. Strain out plant matter and refrigerate. For extra potency, add more powdered cannabis, and cook for another twelve hours.

Notice how oil is used in the recipe for stuffing. In each cannabis is sautéd in butter which extracts the active ingredients. Some people prefer to strain the cannabis butter to remove the plant material. Others leave it in. It is a matter of preference and makes little difference in terms of potency, since the cannabinoids have been transferred from the plant into the oil.

BROWNIE MARY'S CHESTNUT STUFFING

(Serves Six to Eight)

Melt 1 pound of butter or margarine in large frying pan. Add 1/2-3/4 ounce ground cannabis leaf or 2-4 grams of seedless flower and cook 20 minutes covered on low heat, being careful not to burn mixture. Sauté in small amount of olive oil until soft: 3 diced celery stalks, 1 large diced onion, 2 tablespoons minced parsley, 1 teaspoon salt, 1/2 teaspoon poultry seasoning and 1/4 teaspoon pepper. Mix in large bowl: 9 cups stale or packaged bread cubes, 2 slightly beaten eggs and 2 8-ounce cans sliced water chestnuts. Add sautéed vegetables and cannabis-seasoned butter and mix thoroughly with hands. Stuff one 10-12 pound turkey or 2 chickens or 6 pork chops cut 2 inches thick.

Adapted from*Brownie Mary's Marijuana Cookbook/*
Dennis Peron's Recipe For Social Change
Trail of Smoke Publishing Company, 1996

Notice again in the following cookie recipe how the active ingredients are first extracted with butter.

BROWNIE MARY'S CHOCOLATE CHIP COOKIES

(About 60 Cookies)

Melt 1 pound of butter or margarine in double boiler, add 1/2 to 1 ounce ground marijuana leaf or 2-6 grams of seedless flower and cook covered on low heat for 20 minutes, taking care not to burn. Pour the marijuana butter mixture into large bowl. Add 1 cup white sugar, mix well with electric mixer. Add 1 pound brown sugar and mix well. Beat 5 eggs well and mix into sugar mixture. Mix thoroughly. Sift 3 1/2 cups of flour, 2 teaspoons of baking powder and 1 teaspoon salt together, then add to egg/sugar mixture and mix with a large spoon by hand until well-blended. Blend in 2 12-ounce packages of chocolate chips. Mixture will be thick. Drop by teaspoon on 17x11-inch cookie sheet. Bake in oven pre-heated to 375 degrees for 10-12 minutes.

> Adapted from *Brownie Mary's Marijuana Cookbook/*
> *Dennis Peron's Recipe For Social Change*
> *Trail of Smoke Publishing Company, 1996*

ALICE B. TOKLAS' CANNABIS COLD REMEDY

Alice B. Toklas lived from 1877 to 1967 and was the lifelong companion of writer Gertrude Stein as well as being a gourmet cook. In the 1920s and 30s she and Stein regularly hosted the artists and writers of Paris at gatherings that became literary legends. Her cannabis brownies recipe was censored from the American 1954 edition of her cookbook, *The Alice B. Toklas Cookbook.* It did, however, appear in later editions.

Toklas developed the following recipe from the traditional Arabian cannabis food *majoon,* used in Morocco as a folk remedy for warding off the common cold. Toklas describes this Middle Eastern delicacy as a source of "euphoria and brilliant storms of laughter," and cautions that two pieces are "quite sufficient," recommending that they be consumed along with a generous helping of hot mint tea to enhance their effectiveness.

ALICE B. TOKLAS' CANNABIS FRUIT AND NUT BALLS

Chop and mix together about a handful each of stoned dates, dried figs, shelled almonds, and shelled peanuts. Pulverize together in a mortar: 1 teaspoon black peppercorns,1 whole nutmeg, 4 average-size sticks of cinnamon, 1 teaspoon coriander. Separately pulverize about 1/8 ounce cannabis. Melt 1/8 to 1/4 cup (1/2 to 1 stick) butter in pan over low flame. Add powdered cannabis and sauté gently for 5 minutes. Add 1 cup of sugar and stir until dissolved. Add powdered spices to butter mixture and stir until evenly mixed and pour over fruit and nuts. Knead until thoroughly mixed. Make into balls about the size of a walnut.

Adapted from *Shaman Woman, Mainline Lady:*
Women's Writings on the Drug Experience, Quill, New York, 1982.

TIMOTHY LEARY'S CYBER-CULTURE SNACK

This snack, widely known as the "Leary Biscuit," was made popular by Dr. Timothy Leary, the maverick philosopher known more for his quick wit and charm than his kitchen skills.

Early in 1995, Leary was diagnosed with inoperable prostate cancer. He spent the remaining year and a half of his life "designing" his death, saying that "how we die is the most important thing we do." Leary and his cause were popularized on his Internet web site, leary.com, which first gained international popularity for its savvy design, provocative and humorous content, and regular updates on Leary's health as well as his drug intake.

Cooking the biscuit in a microwave oven is an effective and quick way to extract the cannabinoids. As the butter or oil in the cheese heats it melts, sautéing the cannabis which "activates" the THC.

THE LEARY BISCUIT

Take a cracker and add a lump of butter or some cheese (cheddar, Jack or Brie). Top it off with a bud of marijuana. Heat in a microwave oven long enough to melt the cheese or butter, which is also long enough to activate the THC. Serve and enjoy.

Adapted from "The Leary Biscuit" as found on Timothy Leary's website:
www.leary.com by permission of Zach Leary.

EXTRACTING CANNABINOIDS IN WATER

While THC is oil-soluble, there are other medicinally active cannabinoids that are water-soluble. THC is not the only cannabinoid that relieves symptoms; several other cannabinoids have painkilling effects. Preparations containing only water-soluble cannabinoids can therefore be helpful for some conditions, and may be particularly useful when someone desires to avoid the potent psychoactivity associated with THC. Making a tea is a traditional method for extracting water-soluble cannabinoids.

CANNABIS TEA

Place ground cannabis leaves in a teapot, boiling pot, or other container suitable for holding very hot water. Use about 1 teaspoon of cannabis per cup of tea. Pour boiling water over cannabis, using one cup of boiling water per teaspoon of cannabis used. Allow to steep for about 30 minutes. Other favorite teas can be steeped with cannabis to enhance flavor. Tea can be re-heated, or cooled, to desired temperature. If large quantity is made, store in refrigerator.

A variety of enjoyable, therapeutic recipes for cooking with cannabis is abundantly available. One good source is *The Art and Science of Cooking with Cannabis* by Adam Gottlieb. Another is *Marijuana Herbal Cookbook* by Tom Flowers. With experience and experimentation, cooking with cannabis can become a delightful, rewarding pastime as well as an unusually delicious way to administer a beneficial herb.

CHAPTER 10

TINCTURES, OINTMENTS, AND COMPRESSES

Cannabis is a traditional herbal medicine, somewhat unusual among such healing agents for the ubiquity with which smoking has dominated other means of using the herb. Like other beneficial plants, the tradition of cannabis' use spans the full spectrum of methods for processing and administering herbal medicines, including the use of tinctures, salves, poultices, and compresses.

CANNABIS TINCTURES

Tinctures are liquid extracts, usually made with alcohol, containing high concentrations of the active ingredients of beneficial herbs and plants. Tinctures can be added to foods and drinks ingested by placing several drops under the tongue, known as "sublingual" administration, or used topically (on the skin). Tinctures were a widely used means of packaging and administering plant medicines until the end of the nineteenth century, when they faded into relative obscurity with the rise of synthetic drugs and pharmaceutical pills and injections. With the recent renaissance in herbal medicine and homeopathy, however, tinctures are in more widespread use.

ADVANTAGES OF TINCTURES

Cannabis tinctures offer a number of advantages. First of all, they are easily and inexpensively made. Like cannabis foods, the use of tinctures bypasses the health hazards associated with smoking. Where cannabis foods are slow to take effect because the cannabinoids are usually dissolved in oils which take a long time for the body to absorb, cannabis tinctures take effect more rapidly because the alcohol base is more quickly absorbed. But, like the effects of cannabis foods, the effects of tinctures last longer than those of smoking. Tinctures also avoid the dietary concerns of those who wish to limit their intake of fats and oils. Furthermore, cannabis tinctures are usually solutions of alcohol, a preservative which provides long shelf life, unlike oils and fats used in cannabis foods and butters which become rancid, presenting new health hazards.

Whereas a percentage of cannabis' active ingredients are destroyed by heat in the act of smoking, cannabis tinctures make more efficient use of the plant's therapeutic content. Furthermore, cannabis tinctures provide an effective means of using leaves of the plant which may be too low in potency for smoking. Tinctures have the added advantage of being discreet and considerate, avoiding the release of odorous smoke.

Cannabis tinctures are usually made in a solution of alcohol because cannabinoids dissolve fairly readily in alcohol. Since using cannabis tinctures entails the ingestion of small amounts of alcohol, those who avoid alcohol altogether will want to consider eating or smoking instead.

HOW CANNABIS TINCTURES ARE MADE

Making a tincture is simple. Dried or fresh cannabis is finely crumbled or chopped up and submerged in an alcoholic liquid in a glass or stainless steel (never plastic) container with a tight-fitting lid and allowed to sit for two weeks. (See further details below.)

A potent *drinkable* form of alcohol must be used. Rubbing alcohol ("isopropyl" alcohol), can be used to make cannabis extracts suitable for topical application, but is *poisonous when ingested orally*. The alcohol must be at least thirty-proof (sixty percent alcohol content), although it's preferable to use eighty-proof or even stronger alcohol if possible. "Everclear" is an especially potent alcohol product and, therefore, a highly efficient base for potent tinctures. However, it is a specialty item that must often be mail-ordered. The various kinds of vodka from any liquor store will also suffice for this purpose.

One-half to one pint of alcohol is used for every ounce of *dried* cannabis bud, or roughly ten to twenty fluid ounces per ounce of flower bud. A good proportion can be obtained with a small glass jar by filling it two-thirds full with cannabis, and then filling the container to the top with alcohol. Fresh, *undried* bud requires alcohol of a higher proof if possible, and different proportion—five to ten fluid ounces of alcohol solution per one ounce of cannabis. If leaf is used, a tincture of a lower potency will be created unless the ratio of cannabis in the solution is increased. A good rule of thumb for using cannabis leaf is to double the portion of cannabis used for dried bud. In other words, two ounces of dried cannabis for every half-pint to pint of alcohol used. With this ratio, the leaves are crumbled to a very fine mixture in order get completely submerged in the alcohol.

After the alcohol has been added to the cannabis, the container should be covered with a tight-fitting lid and stored in a dark, warm location—around seventy-five degrees Fahrenheit—for about two weeks, during which it is vigorously shaken once or twice a day.

After two weeks, the maximum possible amount of cannabinoids will have been extracted into the liquid from the cannabis. The solid plant matter is strained out of the liquid with a very fine-meshed sieve, cheesecloth, or a coffee filter.

The tincture is poured into a dark tinted bottle (to prevent decomposition of cannabinoids from exposure to light) with a tight-fitting lid. Empty tinted bottles with eyedroppers attached to the lids can be purchased at many health food stores and herbal supply retailers. Use of the dropper facilitates finding, measuring, and maintaining an appropriate dose of the tincture.

Potency of cannabis tinctures varies widely. Appropriate dosage will have to be determined by starting with a few drops, taken directly or added to a beverage, until the desired level of effect is achieved. For a well-extracted cannabis tincture derived from reasonably potent cannabis with a high-proof alcohol beverage, one dropperfull should be the maximum required for a single dose. Adding the tincture to foods may decrease potency to some degree as well as lengthen the amount of time required for results.

TOPICAL APPLICATION

Topical application works through the absorption of medicine through the skin from a compress, salve, or tincture applied directly to the afflicted part of the body. Topical application has been used for arthritis, dermatitis, skin infections, and herpes outbreaks.

There is some debate as to whether cannabinoids are absorbed deeply into the skin when administered topically, as would be desirable, for instance, in the effective treatment of rheumatic joints. But topical application certainly delivers cannabinioids to the surface of the skin, where properties such as anti-infective action are of value. Topical application does not deliver cannabinoids to the central nervous system, and therefore results in no psychoactive high. This aspect of the topical use of cannabis can be an advantage or disadvantage, depending upon the individual and the situation.

Tinctures for oral use can also be used for topical application. Ointments, tinctures made with isopropyl (rubbing) alcohol, and poultices are additional media through which cannabis can be applied topically.

MAKING A CANNABIS OINTMENT

Ointments made with cannabis can be applied directly to the skin. Vaseline serves as an appropriate semi-solid base for a cannabis ointment. Two ounces of Vaseline is simmered together with one-half cup of cannabis butter (a recipe for "cannabutter" can be found in the chapter on cannabis foods) for 15 minutes. Some people prefer to use beeswax instead of Vaseline. The ointment is poured into a container, allowed to cool, then stored at room temperature away from light.

RUBBING ALCOHOL EXTRACT

Chopped or ground cannabis is soaked in isopropyl ("rubbing") alcohol of the kind easily purchased at any corner store. Rules of thumb for proportions are roughly the same as those for making orally ingestable tinctures. The mixture should be steeped in a glass container with a tight-fitting lid away from light until the solution turns a deep green color, which takes about two weeks. The extract so achieved is suitable for topical application only, because *rubbing alcohol is highly toxic* when ingested orally. It can be applied to the troubled area like an ointment. This kind of extract has been applied to help control skin infections and herpes outbreaks, the anti-bacterial and antiviral properties of various cannabinoids working in synergy with the antibacterial properties of rubbing alcohol. With without the plant matter still included in the solution, this kind of extract can also be applied to soothe troubled arthritic joints.

POULTICES AND COMPRESSES

An alternative means of application, taken from folk medicine, is to soak large cannabis leaves in rubbing alcohol for two weeks and then wrap them directly around swollen or inflamed joints or other troubled areas. This is known as a poultice.

Poultices are applied by taking moistened, mashed herbal matter soaked in rubbing alcohol or heated on a stove with a small amount of water, placing it on the skin, and covering it with a cloth compress to hold the poultice in place.

The cloth is heated or cooled by moistening with hot or cold water. Cold poultices are useful for cooling a hot, inflamed area of the body; hot poultices are useful for increasing circulation and relaxing tense or strained muscles.

The cloth with the plant matter underneath it is tied around a troubled joint or limb, or pressed and held against the afflicted area by hand. It can also be held in place by tying an additional piece of cloth around it, which can also be heated or cooled with water of an appropriate temperature.

The herbal matter can be applied indirectly through the cloth, allowing active ingredients to soak their way through the cloth to the skin. Thin cloth made of cotton, which is highly porous, is best for this purpose. In this means of application, the poultice is placed along one side of the moistened cloth, which is then folded over and tied or applied so that the plant material does not directly contact the skin. Alternatively, a first layer of moistened cloth can be applied, covered with herbal matter, and then encased in a second layer of cloth to hold the first layer in place and keep the plant material from falling off the compress. This second layer can also be heated or cooled with water of appropriate temperature to provide insulation and maintenance of the desired temperature.

Using cloth as an intermediate layer between the skin and the medicinal material protects irritated, inflamed, or infected portions of skin from further irritation or abrasion by direct exposure to fragments of plant matter. The cloth, however, may end up absorbing some portion of the desired active ingredients.

Since some important active cannabinoids don't dissolve in water, they won't soak through a water-moistened layer of cloth compress to reach the skin. Presoaking the herbal matter in rubbing alcohol, and adding a certain amount of rubbing alcohol to the water used to moisten the cloth, may be helpful in delivering all the active cannabinoids to the troubled area.

A poultice or compress can be replaced with a fresh one every twenty minutes or so until desired effects are achieved.

While our culture's understanding of cannabis has until recently been dominated by the image of a weed that is smoked to get high, scratching beneath the surface of its history reveals the abundance of methods in and purposes for which this plant is employed as an herbal healing agent. Tinctures were the most common form of cannabis during the heyday of the plant's medicinal application in the nineteenth century, and because of their many advantages, are presently enjoying a resurgence in conjunction with the second historical wave of medicinal use. As the spectrum of the plant's healing potentials continues to be investigated, further uses for topical application, and scientific under-standing of the means by which this and other folk applications are effective, will be forthcoming.

PART THREE

CHAPTER 11

CANNABIS SOOTHES
WHAT AILS YOU

The widespread and long-lived nature of cannabis' medicinal history can be attributed to its unusual qualities. For a medicine of such great potency, cannabis has surprisingly mild physiological impact, a property which minimizes possible complications from its use in treatment. Furthermore, the pathways through which cannabis can be used to serve healing are remarkably diverse and divergent for a single medicine.

THE HISTORY OF CANNABIS MEDICINE

The heyday of cannabis' application in Western medicine took place in the latter half of the nineteenth century. During this period, over one hundred scientific reports were published recommending its use for ailments as diverse as migraines, menstrual problems, and epilepsy. Dr. Solomon H. Snyder, M.D., Professor of Psychiatry and Pharmacology at the Johns Hopkins University School of Medicine, compared the ubiquitousness of cannabis in the late 1900's to that of aspirin today.

Cannabis' popularity in Western medicine declined considerably as the more powerful, more predictable—and more dangerous—opiate derivatives were introduced for the control of pain. Cannabis virtually disappeared from medical practice in the United States after legal impediments to its medical use were first introduced in 1937. The vast database of information on cannabis' medicinal properties accumulated before this government crackdown is still, however, relevant today. In fact, due to the woeful scarcity of systematic investigation into cannabis' healing effects since the 1930s, this material often provides the only documented information about its medicinal uses.

A resurgence of interest in cannabis' healing powers was initiated in 1976, when glaucoma patient Robert Randall won a groundbreaking court case upholding as a "medical necessity" his use of cannabis to maintain his vision. Since then the medicinal value of cannabis and its active ingredients has been the subject of increasing attention, especially in regard to the treatment of glaucoma and the nausea and loss of appetite that accompany cancer chemotherapies and AIDS.

CANNABIS IN THE BODY

The most obvious physiological effect of cannabis is reddening of the eyes due to dilation of the blood vessels. Cannabis stimulates a brief and mild increase in heart rate, comparable to that generated by moderate exercise. The electrical function of the heart, however, is not affected by cannabis.

Cannabis increases blood flow to the brain. This phenomenon results in a two stage response: an initial period of mild stimulation associated with the increase of blood flow to the brain, followed by a period of mild sedation associated with the return of cerebral blood flow to former levels. Some people experience *orthostatic hypotension*, a dizzy feeling caused by a brief, sharp drop in blood pressure that occurs upon standing suddenly. This probably results from changes in physiological functions regulated by the central nervous system through the *vagus* or tenth cranial nerve.

Our understanding of the means by which cannabinoids—the medicinally active components of cannabis—exert their effects can be enhanced by comparison with the somewhat better-understood action of another category of psychoactive substances. The powerful opiate medicines—opium, morphine, codeine, and heroin—accomplish their soothing results by acting upon brain-cell structures called *receptor sites.* Normally, the receptor sites for opiates are activated by natural brain chemicals called endorphins. Endorphins and other *neurotransmitters*— brain hormones involved in the transmission of electrochemical signals along nerve paths—attach themselves to receptor sites on the surfaces of brain cells, initiating metabolic and biochemical changes within the cell and inhibiting or stimulating the release by that cell of further neurotransmitters into the nervous system. The brain changes initiated by endorphins are involved with reducing pain and producing feelings of pleasure and overall physical and mental well-being. Endorphins are the "feel-good" chemicals associated with "runner's high" and the pleasant psychoactive effects of exercise and athletic activity. Our brains release endorphins when we're physically stressed or injured, in the company of loved ones, or performing any activity that we really enjoy.

Endorphin receptors can be imagined as locks, with endorphins acting as keys that unlock good feelings. The chemical structures of morphine and other opiate substances resemble those of the body's native endorphins to a significant degree. This similarity of chemical structure allows opiates to act as "keys" that "open the locks" of endorphin receptors, as if the opiates "fool" the brain into accepting them as its own endorphins. It is this mimicking action that allows opiates to unleash painkilling and pleasure-producing effects similar to those normally created by the endorphins themselves.

Receptor sites have been located in the brain that accept cannabinoids just as endorphin receptors accept opiates. This discovery suggests that the brain naturally manufactures chemicals similar in structure and action to the active ingredients of cannabis. Many of cannabis' effects, therefore, no doubt result from the ability of cannabinoids to mimic the action of brain chemicals that use the same receptor sites. At least one such naturally-occurring neurotransmitter has been discovered. It is called *anandamide,* a name taken from the Sanskrit word *ananda,* which means "spiritual bliss." The functions of anandamide closely resemble the action of THC, one of the primary active ingredients in cannabis. Our understanding of cannabis' therapeutic effects will improve as more of the body's natural cannabinoid-like neurotransmitters and their functions are discovered, perhaps giving rise to new and important medicinal applications for cannabis and its derivatives.

THREE WAYS OF HEALING

Cannabis heals through three primary channels, allowing its healing effects be grouped into three main categories: *palliative* or soothing properties; direct *biological intervention* in the physiology of disease; and beneficial *psychoactive* effects. For most disease conditions, these channels of action interact and overlap, resulting in a healing *synergy*—a total effect that is greater than the sum of its parts.

PALLIATIVE SOOTHING ACTION

A *palliative* medicine is one whose purpose is the relief of suffering. The term "palliative" is derived from the verb palliate, which means to cover over, as in covering over or masking the symptoms of a disease. The commitment of medical practice to alleviate pain and suffering, embodied in the Hippocratic Oath taken by physicians worldwide, has resulted in an entire specialty of health care known as *palliative care* which is concerned not with causes and cures but with the alleviation of symptoms. The aim of palliative care is, quite simply, to make the patient *feel better* by the easing of suffering. A primary objective of palliative care is, therefore, the reduction of pain. Cannabis is often used as a palliative treatment for chronic pain, back pain, and menstrual cramps.

Palliative care can be directed towards easing the suffering created by medical treatments as well as by disease itself. The reduction of nausea among those undergoing chemotherapy for cancer is an example of this kind of palliative care, and is one of cannabis' most outstanding palliative uses.

DIRECT BIOLOGICAL INTERVENTION

When a medicine or other treatment performs *biological intervention,* it acts upon the physiological process of disease, and as a result can slow down or halt the illness' progression. A medicine which eliminates a disease-causing virus, for example, performs a very direct and obvious form of biological intervention. Biological intervention, however, does not necessarily have to address the cause of a disease—which may, after all be unknown—in such a direct manner. Medicines that perform biological intervention may instead interfere with the disease at a point farther along the path of physiological processes that unfold from its initial cause or causes. For instance, a medicine that restores balance to brain chemistry does not necessarily address the reason why the body has produced too much or to little of a brain chemical in the first place, but it may still be an effective treatment for the disease.

Muscle Spasms

Cannabis can have a positive biological impact on movement disorders, epilepsy and other diseases involving muscle spasms and convulsions. Not only can it soothe the pain that accompanies muscle spasms (a palliative effect), but it can *prevent* muscle spasms through a form of biological intervention performed at the centers of motor and muscle control in the nervous system, areas which feature a high distribution of receptor sites at which cannabinoids can bind.

Migraine Headache

Migraine headache is another condition for which cannabis can perform a kind of biological intervention. Part of the disease process of migraine headache involves the release of the neurotransmitter serotonin in the brainstem. THC performs a very precise biological intervention in this aspect of migraine physiology, inhibiting the release of serotonin in the brainstem during migraine attacks but not at other times. (See Chapter 26 for further details.)

Multiple Sclerosis

Cannabis also seems to intervene biologically in the degenerative process of multiple sclerosis (MS). Animal studies have shown that cannabis reduces inflammation of nervous tissue in animals afflicted with an MS-like syndrome, and many MS sufferers report that the use of cannabis has halted, and even reversed, the progression of MS symptoms. More information on MS is in Chapter 17.

BENEFICIAL PSYCHOACTIVE EFFECTS

The soothing psychoactivity of cannabis eases suffering and makes many patients feel a great deal better. In this sense, the cannabis high operates as a powerful *mental* palliative that makes enduring a disease more bearable.

Through its psychoactive properties cannabis opens a pathway of healing that is distinct from and transcends palliative action. Psychoactivity is a way to states of mind useful for healing. It has become increasingly clear that states mind play a major role in resisting and surviving illness as well as in how quickly we recover. Positive mood and outlook, such as that usually engendered by the psychoactivity of cannabis, have a quickening effect on the healing process, creating conditions under which medical treatments work better. Relaxation, optimism, determination, faith, hope, humor, and laughter—all of which are frequently encountered as features of being high— have each been demonstrated to promote physical health and recovery from illness. And, because psychoactivity is fluid in nature—as flexible and malleable as the human mind itself—these properties of cannabis' psychoactivity can be intentionally cultivated and deepened. Focused use of the plant and the practice of various mental and spiritual techniques can channel and intensify the mental changes that cannabis initiates, thereby amplifying their healing power.

HEALING SYNERGY

The three kinds of healing magic that cannabis can be used to perform—palliative, biological, and psychoactive—work in a chorus of harmony, creating a healing synergy.

For instance, a successful *biological* intervention can reduce pain, thereby exerting a valuable *palliative* effect. Psychoactivity can soothe the mind and make people feel better, thereby exerting a psychologically *palliative* effect.

Palliative pain reduction can liberate the mind from preoccupation with pain, bringing about a change in mind-state that is a form of *psychoactive* effect. Changes in mind-state induced by psychoactivity can bolster immune function, thereby exerting positive *biological* impact.

Palliative effects, in reducing pain, also reduce tension and stress. Stress reduction can favorably alter biochemistry and empower immunity, a route whereby *palliative* action can have positive *biological* consequences.

These examples of the synergy that can occur between the three kinds of healing magic characteristic of cannabis highlight how each type of healing action can flow into, nourish, and amplify the next, generating an upward spiral that lifts towards healing.

MEDICAL CONDITIONS BENEFITED

Conditions covered in the following section range from common, everyday troubles suffered by all of us at one time or other, like back pain or nausea, to more severe conditions like cancer, multiple sclerosis, and AIDS. The discussions demonstrate the interplay of the palliative, biological, and psychoactive effects of cannabis in specific disease conditions.

If the specific condition about which one is concerned does not appear in the following chapters, it might be useful to scan through the coverage of the maladies that have causes or symptoms similar to those of illnesses of specific interest. Cannabis may be of value in such cases if it has proven useful for a similar or related conditions. If you think cannabis might be helpful for your condition or that of a loved one, always consult your doctor or other qualified health practitioner before attempting to integrate cannabis into the treatment program.

CHAPTER 12

ARTHRITIS

Arthritis is a disease that affects the joints and the surrounding tissues, including muscles, membrane linings, and cartilage. The body's efforts to overcome the condition result in painful inflammation—heat, swelling, pain, redness of skin, and tenderness—in the affected areas. Although the cause of arthritis is not known, it is thought to be an *automimmune* disorder—a condition in which an immune system gone haywire attacks the body's own tissues.

Arthritis is three times as common among women as men. The onset usually occurs between ages twenty and sixty, with the highest incidence between ages thirty-five and forty-five. The range of seriousness of arthritis is considerable. In the worst cases severe arthritis can result in permanent disfigurement or crippling.

MEDICAL TREATMENTS FOR ARTHRITIS

There is no cure for arthritis yet. However, with early detection, physical therapy, use of pain-relieving and anti-inflammatory drugs like aspirin, and drugs that alter the immune response like cortisone, disability can usually be prevented. Cortisone-type drugs, which can provide dramatic relief of pain for short periods, unfortunately decrease in effectiveness when used over time. The side effects of cortisone and related medicines can be hazardous: increase or decrease of appetite, nausea, restlessness and insomnia, dizziness, headache, thirstiness, increased frequency of urination, depression and mood swings, irregular heartbeat, pain, and menstruation problems.

CANNABIS AND ARTHRITIS

The ancient Roman natural historian Pliny the Elder, writing in the first century B.C.E., recommended the use of cannabis for relief of arthritis. A European *Treatise On Hemp* held that a poultice made from boiled cannabis root "softens and restores the joints or fingers or toes that are dried or shrunk," noting that such a preparation is also "very good against the gout, and other humours that fall upon the nervous, muscular, or tendinous parts." Contemporary Jamaican folk healers use poultices made from the flowering buds and leaves of cannabis. And in 1994, the *Times* (of London) reported that "the demand for cannabis among British pensioners has stunned doctors, police and suppliers....The old people use the drug to ease the pain of such ailments as arthritis and rheumatism. Many are running afoul of the law for the first time in their lives as they try to obtain supplies."

Several cannabinoids have both *analgesic* (pain-relieving) and anti-inflammatory effects, a combination particularly helpful for arthritic people. Cannabidiol (CBD), one of the main active ingredients in cannabis, has been found to be as effective an anti-inflammatory agent as aspirin. Since arthritis appears to be an autoimmune disorder, additional relief for arthritis may be provided by cannabis modulating the body's immune responses.

Cannabis can be smoked or eaten to relieve the general pain, inflammation, and discomfort characteristic of arthritis. Cannabis poultices can be applied topically to troubled areas. How to prepare and use cannabis poultices is described in Chapter 10, Tinctures, Ointments, and Compresses.

CHAPTER 13

ASTHMA

Asthma is a condition characterized by attacks of wheezing and shortness of breath that starts with spasms in the involuntary muscles surrounding the air passages in the lungs that constrict the passageways. In milder asthma, only the larger air passageways, or *bronchi*, are affected. In more severe asthma, either the bronchi or the smaller air passageways, called *bronchioles*, may be involved.

During an asthma attack a lot of mucus is produced which is difficult to cough up because of the constriction of air passageways which leads to buildup of mucus further blocking the passageways, making it even more difficult for the person to get air. Then the mucus-generating membranes lining the passageways become swollen, causing further blocking. Eventually it becomes a vicious cycle of spasms constricting air passages, mucus buildup, and swelling of mucus tissue making it increasingly difficult to get enough oxygen and possibly leading to a medical emergency.

Asthma afflicts about ten million Americans and is fatal to about four thousand people every year. It occurs more frequently among children than adults. Childhood asthma usually dissipates on its own as the person grows older, but adult onset asthma generally doesn't improve without treatment.

The cause of asthma is not known. However, the triggers of asthma attacks fall into four categories. Attacks can be triggered by exposure to a substance to which the person is allergic, such as pollen, dust or feathers. Bronchitis or infection of lung tissue can precipitate asthma attacks. Another trigger is "primary irritation," caused by fog, hot or cold air, exposure to smoke, aerosols, chemical fumes, and sharp changes in weather. A fourth trigger is emotional upset such as frustration, worry, and stress.

MEDICAL TREATMENTS FOR ASTHMA

Among children, simple antihistamines are sometimes all that's required to quell an asthma attack. Stronger pharmecutical treatments for asthma include bronchodilators, which are inhaled from special dispensers the moment an asthma attack begins or taken in tablet form. Bronchodilators relax bronchial muscles and widen air passages in the lungs.

Unfortunately bronchodilators sometimes cause anxiety, insomnia, and nausea and have been associated with many deaths among asthma sufferers. In more severe cases of asthma, bronchodilators are inadequate, and may have to be combined with other treatments if they are to work at all. Drugs called *corticosteroids* are often used on a preventive basis for severe asthma. Corticosteroids suppress allergic reactions and reduce inflammation and swelling in bronchial passageways, helping to prevent asthma attacks and allowing bronchodilators to be effective if attacks do take place.

Corticosteroids can be used only for short term intervention because ongoing use can lead to serious side effects. Corticosteroids can cause insomnia, anxiety, and nausea, other side effects include abdomenal or back pain, fatigue, weakness, shortness of breath, dizziness and fainting, fast, hard, or irregular heatbeat, and loss of appetite and weight. Corticosteroids can cause impairment of vision, increase in blood pressure, thirstiness, and menstrual problems, they weaken immuity, particularly susceptibility to infections in the lungs or mouth, and cause dependence. Their use also features the development of tolerance, meaning that larger doses have to be used over time for the medication to remain effective.

CANNABIS AND ASTHMA

Scientific study has shown that THC relieves bronchial constriction in asthma sufferers, and permits a freer flow of air through the lungs of people who do not have asthma. THC relieves muscle spasms, including soothing bronchial muscle spasms that initiate asthma attacks. Cannabis preparations have antiallergic properties which can be beneficial for asthma sufferers whose attacks are triggered by allergns.

Studies have compared both THC in smoked form and in an aerosol spray to the efficacy of medical bronchodilators. THC showed either equal or lesser peak effects and the soothing effects of THC did not kick in as quickly as those of pharmeceuticals, but the THC effects lasted longer. THC presents considerably less risk than do medical bronchodilators, and apparently works through a different mechanism.

Smoking cannabis as a treatment for asthma presents obvious health risks. Long-term, heavy smoking of cannabis can produce bronchitis, a condition which can trigger attacks in asthma sufferers. Cannabis smoke contains tars, carcinogens, and other substances that are toxic to the lungs and the tiny hair-like cells (*cilia*) that help the lungs to manage the flow of mucus. The antiasthmatic effect of orally-ingested THC has been shown to be less reliable, and to be slower to take effect than when cannabis is smoked or when THC is administered in an aerosol spray.

Research using aerosol THC for asthma has been found to provide reliable benefits without adverse side effects. Aerosol concentrations of THC sufficient for antiasthmatic action were found to have negligible psychoactivity and effect on heart rate. Researchers who found that aerosol-administered THC was irritating to the lungs suspected that they had used an aerosol with unnecessarily high concentrations of this cannabinoid. Future research may find that other cannabinoids in aerosol form are even more effective than THC, and even less irritating to lung tissue. Aerosol sprays containing THC or other cannabinoids are not commercially available, but may be the wave of the future regarding cannabis-related treatment for asthma.

Until such products become available, people who wish to use cannabis for asthma may find tinctures of cannabis to be the best option. Tinctures do not irritate the lungs, and have faster action than cannabis prepared in foods.

CHAPTER 14

BACK PAIN

Chronic lower back pain is often associated with muscle spasms. Office workers, who form a large share of the work force, often have to maintain the same posture seated behind a desk for hours, day after day, using office furniture whose poor design strains the muscular system, particularly the lower back. This kind of lifestyle promotes a high incidence of back pain and spasms not only because of this physical factor, but because it is stressful in many other ways. Stress stimulates muscle tension, leading to the kind of muscular rigidity that can cause pain in the back and other areas of the body. Furthermore, there's a higher propensity to have muscle spasms when very stressed.

Cannabis provides some people with relief from severe and chronic back pain and the muscle spasms associated with it, often working where other therapies have failed. Cannabis appears to affect several different sites in order to provide this soothing relief. Cannabinoids bind to receptors in spinal motor neurons, skeletal muscles, and at the the junctions between nerves and muscles, all areas where they could act to help restore healthy posture, normal movements, and muscle tone. Some chiropractors have been known to recommend cannabis to their patients for this indication in states where it is legal to do so. One elderly man always eats a cannabis cookie before boarding an airplane; besides relieving anxiety about flying, it prevents him from developing the lower back pain that he had previously come to associate with long stretches of time spent confined in airplane seating.

CHAPTER 15

CHRONIC PAIN

Chronic pain can result from a wide variety of conditions and situations and is one of the most difficult problems for health practitioners to treat. It often follows many kinds of surgery, as well as injuries from incidents like car accidents and athletic mishaps. It can even spring from certain types of hormone problems, and may occur as a side effect of various medications. People who have relatively common and simple problems like flat feet from fallen arches may experience chronic pain, and chronic pain also goes along with many of the conditions discussed in this chapter, from AIDS and cancer to arthritis and back trouble. Severe and chronic pain can have its own side effects like hot and cold sweat, nausea, and vomiting. People are most likely to have such reactions to "breakthrough pain," when ongoing pain spikes up to especially high levels.

CONVENTIONAL TREATMENT FOR CHRONIC PAIN

Conventional medicine treats chronic pain with opiate-type medicines such as codeine, which present many problems, foremost among which is high addictiveness. Furthermore, opiates feature rapid development of tolerance, which means that the dosages have to be increased as time goes by. As the dose goes up, so does the severity of addiction, and therefore the withdrawal symptoms experienced when the medication is stopped also intensifies. If the medication is discontinued, the underlying pain reappears and the intense physical discomfort that accompanies opiate withdrawal is added to the suffering.

Much addiction and general drug use has its roots in pain. Some people who are habitual users of street opiates may have first become addicted when they were treated with morphine in a hospital. Many street drug habits originated with a car accident or other injury that left the person in severe chronic pain. This kind of behavior is known as "self-medication".

The side effects of opiate painkillers tend to increase along with the dosage used. For instance, many people using opiates for chronic pain find that the dosages required for adequate pain relief leave them feeling so "doped up" that they can't function. This effect occurs because these drugs result in an overall decrease in both physical and mental sensation, often leaving people woozy, tired, and incapable of thinking clearly.

Non-addictive painkillers are also used to treat chronic pain. The problem with these is that they are rarely strong enough to provide adequate pain relief.

CANNABIS AND CHRONIC PAIN

Comparing the way cannabis and its derivatives function as pain-killers to the manner in which opiate-type pain relievers work yields a stark and illuminating contrast. First of all, cannabis is generally considered non-addictive and doesn't lead to severe withdrawal symptoms, if any. Furthermore, like the psychoactive and other effects of cannabis, tolerance doesn't develop to cannabis' painkilling effects. The psychoactivity of cannabis is far less debilitating, if at all, and if any problems do arise in this area they can usually be easily mastered over time. Some patients who felt that their prescription opiates made them withdraw into a stuporous haze have reported being more functional, alert, and competent when they switched to an amount of cannabis that killed their pain just as effectively.

The painkilling properties of THC have been scientifically compared to those of codeine and other commonly-used painkillers. THC was found to be as effective as codeine in relieving pain. Furthermore, the dose of THC required to kill pain effect turned out to be far smaller than the amount of codeine required to give the same level of relief. Cannabis has also been shown to have far fewer physical side effects than commonly-used painkillers at dosages that have equally soothing effects.

Scientific studies have provided even more exciting news about the painkilling effects of cannabis: The same dosage of cannabis has a consistently *stronger* painkilling effect for experienced users of cannabis than for inexperienced users. This means that tolerance to cannabis' pain-soothing properties doesn't build up, so that people who are using cannabis for pain won't have to use more and more over time. For some users *less* cannabis can be used to achieve the same degree of soothing after they have used it for some time. The reason for this apparent anomoly has to do with learning. The first few times people get "stoned" they usually experience body and senses anew, almost as if for the first time. Rubber legs, where one feels unable to walk without wobbling, is a common experience along with becoming transfixed by vivid sounds and colors, giggling uncontrollably and craving sweets, for example. These novel sensations along with an uplift in mood, optimistic outlook, and openness are stimulated by cannabis' psychoactive properties. With subsequent use heightened senses become more familiar. Eventually, a small amount of cannabis can serve to trigger psychoactive responses learned in earlier trips.

A single dose of cannabis can relieve pain for several hours. The larger the dose, the longer the pain-relieving effect will last. At higher doses, THC, one of the main active ingredients in cannabis, acts as a sedative as well. This sedative effect can help soothe the tension that often accompanies being in pain.

HOW CANNABIS RELIEVES PAIN

The body's native opiate-like chemicals, known as *endorphines* and *enkephalins* are an important aspect of the body's management of pain. These chemicals bind to receptor sites on certain types of nerve cells, inducing a "feel-good" state. They also affect the transmission of pain signals through the nervous system, changing the person's experience of the pain and its felt intensity. Opiate drugs bind to the same receptor sites used by the body's native painkilling chemicals, and work similarly.

Receptors also exist in the nervous system for cannabinoids, and at least one of the native chemicals that use these receptors has been discovered. This substance, *ananadamide,* has effects on physiology and consciousness nearly identical to those of THC. It is possible that the body's natural cannabinoid systems—its cannabinoid-like chemicals and the nerve cells with which they interact—accompany the endorphin system as important parts of the body's natural ways of dealing with pain.

HOW TO USE CANNABIS TO RELIEVE PAIN

There are a number of strategies for using cannabis to treat pain. It can be used by itself on an as-needed basis, in dosages that change according to the level of pain. It can also be used effectively with or alternating with over-the-counter painkillers. Furthermore, the use of cannabis and opiates for pain is not necessarily an either-or issue. If cannabis is used in an ongoing regimen of medication, opiates could be added or substituted during periods when pain levels rise to breakthrough levels. Conversely, if opiates are being used as the basis of the ongoing regimen, cannabis could be added when breakthrough pain occurs. This strategy could help prevent higher levels of opiates having to be used during breakthrough periods. If higher doses of opiates were used for breakthrough instead of cannabis, the person's tolerance to the opiates would tend to increase, creating a situation in which their baseline dose of opiates would have to remain higher even after the breakthrough pain period was over.

Another practical consideration in the use of cannabis for pain is whether smoking or eating is better. Donald, a student in photography, had severe chronic pain and limited range of motion in his neck after a car accident, which interfered with studying. Sitting at a desk and reading and writing involved especially uncomfortable postures for him. The problem was so bad that he enrolled in a special program for disabled students which allowed him to complete coursework at a slower rate than was generally required. During the eight years following the accident he tried many therapies and pain medications, but his pain was no better. He still hadn't finished school, and, since there seemed no hope that he would be able to do so, he commenced making arrangements to drop out. As this was happening, he decided to try cannabis for his problem through a doctor and a buyer's club.

Smoking cannabis offered little relief of his pain. However, he found that eating cannabis-containing foods provided nearly miraculous relief. His pain declined to managable levels, and the range of motion his his head, neck and shoulders loosened tremendously. He was able to stay in school, and completed his degree within a year and a half of his beginning to use cannabis.

CHAPTER 16

DEPRESSION

Depression is a state of mind characterized by continuing feelings of pessimism, hopelessness, despair, loss of interest in life, boredom, and sadness. Symptoms of depression include insomnia or excessive sleeping, loss of appetite or overeating, decreased sex drive, constipation, difficulty with concentrating and with making decisions, and irritability. Depressed people may experience bodily pains, such as headaches or chest pains, that have no medical explanation. People suffering from depression may have long fits of unexplained weeping, tend to isolate themselves socially, and may be plagued by exaggerated feelings of guilt and thoughts of suicide. Foremost among the symptoms of depression are listlessness and chronic tiredness, symptoms beneath which depression may mask itself. People who feel "tired all the time" may actually be suffering from depression.

Winston Churchill, the celebrated British statesman and Prime Minister of England during World War II, suffered from depression. He called it "the black dog." Once when yet another bout of depression had started to take hold of him, he recorded in his journal, "the black dog is once again upon me."

Episodes of depression can last from a few days to several years. Long, severe bouts of depression are considered psychiatric disorders. In its most severe form, depression can appear as a catatonic-like state.

Depression can be triggered by various life stresses and disruptive events. Loss is a frequent trigger of depression, such as the breakup of a marriage or the death of a loved one as well as loss of a job, money, or a place to live. Major surgery, severe illness, and disability can trigger depression. Significant life transitions like change of job, retirement, menopause, or moving to a new area can precipitate depression.

Depression can occur as a side effect of medications, such as those used to treat high blood pressure and tranquilizers. Depression can be a symptom of physical illnesses, including hormonal problems, diabetes, and pancreatic cancer.

Sometimes depression has no visible cause. In such cases it is thought to result from an imbalance of brain chemistry.

This form of depression is called "endogenous" depression, meaning "generated from within." Low levels of the brain chemicals serotonin, dopamine, and norepinephrine have all been implicated in endogenous depression.

MEDICAL TREATMENTS FOR DEPRESSION

A vast armamentarium of antidepressant medications has been steadily increasing since they were first marketed in the 1950s. By the 1990's, the most popular category of antidepressant in the United States was *selective serotonin reuptake inhibitors* (SSRIs), such as Prozac, Zoloft, Paxil, and Effexor which boost levels of the mood-modulating brain chemical serotonin by preventing its reabsorption into brain cell storage areas. Some SSRIs also effect the activity of norepinephrine, an excitatory brain chemical.

Fifty to seventy percent of patients using serotonin reuptake inhibitors achieve adequate results. However, they may have side effects which can include nausea, headache, loss of appetite and weight loss, agitation, loss of sex drive and difficulty in having orgasm. Fortunately most of the side effects are transitory.

Before the advent of serotonin reuptake drugs, the most commonly used antidepressants were tricyclics. The effectiveness rate of tricyclics is about the same as that of SSRIs. Side effects of tricyclics include dizziness, dry mouth, blurred vision, constipation, difficulty urinating, weight gain, problems with sexual function, and orthostatic hypotension—a brief, sharp drop in blood pressure upon standing up suddenly that causes a momentary dizziness. These side effects tend to last longer than those of the SSRIs. Another danger is that tricyclics increase heart rate and can disturb the rhythm of the heart, posing risks for patients with cardiovascular problems.

Another type of antidepressants commonly used is Monamine Oxidase Inhibitors (MAOIs), which work by inhibiting the action of monamine oxidase, the enzyme that initiates the metabolic breakdown of serotonin, norepinephrine, and dopamine—all brain chemicals that play an important role in mood. By interfering with the action of this enzyme MAOIs elevate mood by increasing the levels of serotonin, norepinephrine, and dopamine active in the nervous system.

The effectiveness of MAOIs is significantly higher than that of tricyclics and SSRIs. However, careless use can lead to severe side effects. A person using MAOIs who eats certain aged cheeses, red wine, or sufficient quantities of other foods containing the amino acid tyramine, may experience the "cheese effect" which is a sharp, sudden, and potentially dangerous increase in blood pressure which in extreme cases can result in fatal brain hemorrhaging. Other side effects of MAOIs include constipation, weight gain, orthostatic hypotension, insomnia, and difficulty in achieving orgasm for men. Aside from the cheese effect, the other side effects of MAOIs tend to be transitory. Because of the cheese effect, MAOIs are usually used only after other drugs have failed.

CANNABIS AND DEPRESSION

About thirty percent of patients with depression either respond poorly to antidepressants or find the side effects intolerable. For these people cannabis may be a viable alternative. A significant difference between cannabis and antidpressant medications is that the mood-lifting effects of cannabis are experienced within a few minutes after smoking it or about an hour after ingesting. The mood-changing effects of pharmeceutical antidepressants, on the other hand, usually take several days or weeks to kick in.

As early as 1845, cannabis was prescribed for obsessive rumination, worrying, and melancholia, as doctors called depression in those times. Smoking cannabis usually has a soothing effect that helps one to relax and set worries aside.

From 1845 to 1973, many studies explored the possible value of cannabis and THC in the treatment of mood disorders, including depression, with inconclusive results. In 1947, just before the advent of the first pharmeceutical antidepressants, an English doctor administered synthetic THC to fifty depressed patients and reported improvement in thirty-six of them. Subsequent studies comparing the effects of THC to placebo in depressed patients have not produced comparably positive results.

Depression is often part of debilitating, challenging, and life-threatening diseases, particularly terminal cases. The self-medication of mild to moderate depression underlies a great deal of nonperscription cannabis use. The psychoactive properties in cannabis have an uplifting influence on mood; after smoking it people feel more cheerful and optimistic. Cannabis can enhance the impact of mental exercises designed to alter mood and outlook. The psychoactive properties produce a high in in the user which is just what a depressed person who feels "low" needs. Imaging positive possibilities, thinking of alternatives and being optimistic counter depression and are easier to do when high on cannabis. Depressed people usually feel hopeless and stuck and become myopic, unable to see alternatives. Cannabis stimulates creativity, making it easier to view things from a different perspective.

Good communication with family and friends is a factor that both relieves and prevents depression. Cannabis itself tends to generate feelings of empathy and can open doorways to interpersonal communication which is why people like to share a joint. It makes them feel more friendly and outgoing. Smoking cannabis with a caregiver or friend can generate feelings of acceptance and belonging which are counterpoised to the feelings of alienation and isolation that come with depression and disease.

Depression mutes feelings and sensations. Depressed people fail to appreciate, or even notice, much of what would ordinarily give them pleasure such as the company of friends and loved ones, the sounds of lovely music, the beauty of natural environments or of works of art, the humor of a good joke. The feelings of social connectedness, sensory enhancement, and stimulation of humor associated with the psychoactivity of cannabis can help a depressed person reactivate the senses.

Numerous personal testimonies relate stories in which cannabis has provided welcome and reliable relief from depression where standard medications failed or produced troublesome side effects. Cannabis' soothing and uplifting effects can be particularly helpful in cases of depression marked by irritability and pessimism. Cannabis' appetite-stimulating effect is helpful in depression with loss of appetite. People who use cannabis after having suffered depression for years report that it helps them to push back depressing thoughts and to enjoy the beauty of the world anew.

Cannabis can be helpful as a mood-stabilizing medicine for those whose depression is accompanied by episodes of *mania*—highly energized periods characterized by excessive stimulation, extreme euphoria, inability to sleep, and wild mood swings including fits of rage.

Changes in consciousness brought about by the interaction of cannabis with other psychoactives can be unpredictable. Patients using prescription psychiatric medication should be cautious about experimenting with cannabis and do so only under medical supervision. Cannabis might be especially useful as an occasional or ongoing adjunct to conventional medications with which it turns out to be compatible.

CHAPTER 17

EPILEPSY

Epilepsy refers to a variety of brain malfunctions that cause sei-zures ranging from a few moments of being "spaced out" to sudden changes in personality and behavior, to the intense spasmodic fits or convulsions of grand mal epilsepsy, the most well-known form of the disease. Medicines used to control epileptic episodes include Dilantin and barbiturates, the latter having high addictive potential. These medicines don't generally succeed completely. Furthermore, they can cause severe negative reactions, from emotional disturbances like de-pression to bone softening and anemia.

The convulsions characteristic of grand mal epilepsy are violent muscle spasms. Cannabis has been demonstrated to be particularly effective in controlling muscle spasms. In fact, cannabis has been used as an anticonvulsant since ancient times in India, and was widely employed for this purpose by nineteenth century Western medical practitioners.

Tod Mikuriya, M.D., a leading medical marijuana expert, noted that a 1949 article buried in a journal of chemical abstracts reported that a substance related to THC controlled epileptic seizures in a group of children more effectively than diphenylhydantoin (Dilantin), a com-monly prescribed anticonvulsant. Dilantin is still one of the most common antiepileptics. Recent research suggests that cannabis—par-ticularly cannabidiol (CAD), one of its active ingredients—can be useful for grand mal epilepsy patients as an adjunct to conventional medications. Patients can reduce their dosages of prescribed medicines when they add cannabidiol to their treatment. In some cases, epileptic episodes disappear completely.

CHAPTER 18

GLAUCOMA

Glaucoma is a leading cause of blindness resulting from a build up of pressure inside the eyeball. In glaucoma the *intraocular pressure* inside the eye is abnormally high because the eye creates too much fluid, or the passageways through which the fluid flows out of the eye are blocked.

CANNABIS LEGAL FOR GLAUCOMA

In 1972 Robert Randall was diagnosed with inoperable glaucoma, with the prediction that he had three to five years of remaining sight. Randall used all the available glaucoma medications at the highest permissible doses, but his condition continued to worsen just as his doctor had predicted. Then one night, when he smoked cannabis for the first time in more than a year, he noticed that the optical halos, one of his primary symptoms, were absent from his vision. For the first time in years Randall felt hopeful that his sentence to a life of blindness was not fixed. He began experimenting with cannabis with very positive results.

Randall made it a personal mission to obtain cannabis legally to treat his glacuoma. To prepare his case for the government he underwent two lengthy, extensive, highly controlled medical experiments at the Jules Stein Eye Institute at UCLA and the Wilmer Eye Institute at Johns Hopkins University. Both of these respected scientific institutions reached the conclusion that he would go blind if deprived of cannabis. Eventually Randall won a groundbreaking case to became the first person to gain legal, medically supervised access to cannabis since the 1930s. Twenty-five years later, in 1997, Robert Randall could still see.

TREATMENT AND MISTREATMENT

The medical treatment for glaucoma is eyedrops containing drugs called beta-blockers. While these are often very effective, they can cause depression, exacerbate asthma, decrease the heart rate, and increase the danger of heart failure. Eyedrops containing epinephrine can also be effective. But they, too have negative side effects of irritation to the white of the eye and possibly aggravating high blood pressure or heart disease. Drugs that contract the pupil, such as pilocarpine are used less frequently because they can cause cataracts and actually impair vision rather than preserve it.

The most common form of glaucoma, called *open angle* glaucoma, afflicts about a million Americans. In open angle glaucoma, the channels that carry fluid out of the eyeball gradually become narrower and narrower causing the intraocular pressure to increase slowly over time, damaging the optic nerve that relays signals from the eye to the brain and resulting in blindness. Fortunately, it can be treated with cannabis.

Cannabis relieves symptoms by reducing intraocular pressure, thereby slowing down the progress of the condition and sometimes bringing it to a complete halt. The pressure-reducing effects achieved by using cannabis last for an average of four to five hours.

Use of cannabis by glaucoma patients does not interfere with their visual acuity or eye function and incurs no damage to the structures of the eye. Furthermore, tolerance to cannabis' pressure-reducing effects does not develop, which means that the quantity used does not have to be increased over time as is the case with so many medicines.

Many glaucoma patients cannot use standard drug treatments because of the severity of side effects they experience. Cannabis, on the other hand, presents no known risks or discomforts in the treatment of glaucoma remotely resembling in magnitude the problems often presented by the standard medical treatments. Furthermore, cannabis has succeeded in containing the progress of glaucoma in many cases where other medications have offered little promise of hope. How cannabis reduces eyeball pressure, specifically, is not understood but it is generally believe that it works through a different mechanism than conventional treatments.

As many as fifty percent of glacuoma patients cannot tolerate the side effects of conventional medicines! Cannabis has so few negative side effects that its use is almost always indicated when conventional medicine has failed and when surgery is too dangerous. People suffering from "end-stage" glaucoma where most vision has already been lost and blindness is on the way may also find relief with cannabis. Robert Randall, who was at the end stage when he began using cannabis, has been able to maintain his sight for twenty-five years.

Marinol, a prescription pharmaceudical which contains THC, one of the most active ingredients in cannabis, comes in pill form and is effective in reducing intraocular pressure. Most galcuoma patients, however, prefer smoking to the pills. Smoking small amounts of cannabis six to ten times a day is good a way of "titrating the dose," a term doctors use for determining the smallest effective dose.

CHAPTER 19

INSOMNIA

Sleep disorders are so widespread in our society as to form the basis of an industry so vast that the variety of prescription, over-the-counter, herbal, nutritional, and other remedies available to the consumer amounts to hundreds, perhaps thousands, of products. Problems with sleep are especially prevalent among the elderly, a population that therefore accounts for a very large share of prescriptions for "heavy artillery" sleep aids—barbiturates, like phenobarbital, and benzodiazepines, like Halcion.

Problems with these conventional *hypnotics,* as sleep-inducing medications are called, include rapid development of tolerance so that higher and higher doses are required to achieve the same level of effectiveness, "rebound insomnia" in which the sleep disorder may be intesified when the medication is discontinued, high incidence of addictive difficulties, and the possibility of lethal or at least coma-inducing overdoses. In fact, *Webster's New World Dictionary* refers to barbiturates as "dangerous, habit-forming depresssants."

CANNABIS AND INSOMNIA

Cannabis, and the other hand, can be an effective sleep aid and features none of the complications encountered with pharmaceuticals. In 1890, British physician J.R. Reynolds, M.D., recommended cannabis for "senile insomnia" a sleep problems associated with aging, noting that use of cannabis could remain effective for years without producing tolerance.

Among the constituents of cannabis, cannabidiol (CBD) has been isolated as an ingredient likely to be responsible for a large part of its sedative effects. (THC, it is now believed, is more associated with the initial period of stimulation that follows the ingestion of cannabis.) A five week long controlled study which tested the efficacy of CBD as a sleep aid among a group of fifteen insomniacs revealed that "sleep quality was significantly influenced by...cannabidiol as two-thirds of the subjects slept more than seven hours...Most subjects had few interruptions of sleep and reported having a good night's sleep."

In addition to the side effects and complications linked to prescription sleep medicines, most of them are also associated with kidney problems. Cannabis, however, does not cause stress to the kidneys because its active ingredients are not water-soluble but are oil- or fat-soluble and not processed through the kidneys. Tod Mikuriya, M.D., has pointed out that our country's growing population of elderly people would stand to receive special benefit from the broader application of cannabis and its derivatives as aids to sleep. They are significantly more prone to kidney problems and failure than the population at large. No doubt a large number of kidney problems among elders could be prevented if cannabis or its derivatives were used as substitute sleep aids in cases where they proved to be sucessful.

Differing strains of cannabis may exhibit widely variant levels of efficacy as sleep aids. The action of cannabis is characterized by an initial period of stimulation followed by a (usually longer) period of sedation. Some strains of cannabis feature stimulant properties significantly stronger than their sedative effects; in other strains this balance is reversed. Determinant factors in this variance may be the ratios and concentrations of THC (associated with stimulation) and CBD (linked to sedation), as well as the levels and proportions of the over sixty other cannabinoids that can be present in the herb.

CHAPTER 20

MENSTRUAL CRAMPS

Menstrual cramps, medically known as "dysmenorrhea" and called "the cramps" by most women, are pains in the abdomen, lower back, thighs accompanied by bloating. The ancient Chinese used cannabis to treat menstrual cramps. Cannabis tinctures were commonly prescribed in the Nineteenth Century for relief from this malady. Doctors writing at that time extolled its virtues, saying that it was the most reliable means available for relieving the discomfort of cramps and that no other medicine gave such good results. With the advent of more modern pain relievers and legal restrictions on the use of cannabis, this knowledge was practically forgotten.

Since the 1960s, modern women who first used Cannabis recreationally have rediscovered its soothing benefits for this problem. The herb has become the treatment of choice for many of them. Cannabis is often used for menstrual cramps in conjunction with over-the-counter painkillers such as ibuprofen with good results.

CHAPTER 21

MIGRAINE HEADACHES

Migraine headaches are severe, long-lasting, recurring headaches, often accompanied by nausea and vomiting. Throbbing pain located on one side of the head, above or behind one eye is a distinctive characteristic of the migraine.

People suffering from the classic migraine experience a neurological warning of the impending attack called an *aura*. Auras include numbness and tingling in the limbs; strange visual events, like flashes of light, blind spots, or wavy lines; and mental disruptions like disorientation, confusion, and difficulty putting thoughts into words. Migraines can be debilitating, not only because they are so painful, but because the level of pain can rise sharply in response to lights, sounds, and physical activity, leaving the sufferer with little choice but to remain in bed in a dark, quiet room until the worst has passed.

The incidence of migraines in our society is on the rise. One in five people have experienced at least one migraine. Women are much more likely to get them than men.

It is believed that dilation of blood vessels to the scalp and the brain cause migraines, which tend to be associated with stress and tension, fatigue, menstruation, use of birth control pills or alcohol, and from eating certain foods to which the person has a bad reaction. Changes in the level of a brain chemical called serotonin have been linked to migraines.

The ancient Egyptians smoked the leaves of the cannabis plant for headaches. For many physicians in the nineteenth century, cannabis was the preferred treatment for headaches, especially migraines. Popularity of treating headaches with cannabis declined when younger doctors turned to injectable opiates after the invention of the syringe in the 1850s because they were enthused by the speed of relief achieved by injection. No one anticipated the addiction problems that resulted.

Modern opiate-type drugs, such as Demerol, are still commonly used for migraines. Thorazine, a tranquilizer used to treat psychosis, is also used. These drugs soothe the pain of migraines when they have started. Drugs to control blood pressure are taken on an ongoing basis by chronic migraine sufferers to *prevent* attacks from occurring, including beta-blockers, calcium channel blockers, and Propanolol. Ironically, some of these medications can cause chronic tension headaches—which seems to defeat the purpose of treating migraines! Ten to twenty percent of migraine sufferers get little or no help from such treatments.

CANNABIS AND MIGRAINES

Cannabis soothes the intense pain associated with migraine and helps relieve nausea and vomiting. Even better news for migraine sufferers, however, is that cannabis, if taken at the first sign of an attack, can sometimes cut it short or prevent it, which is amazing since migraine attacks can otherwise last for as long as three days! Cannabis, like the blood pressure medicines mentioned, can be used on an ongoing basis as a preventive measure.

Recent scientific investigation indicates that THC, one of the main active ingredients in cannabis, affects the release of serotonin, the brain chemical linked to migraines. Interestingly, THC has this effect *only* during migraine attacks, and not at other times. The way cannabis works to soothe and even halt migraine attacks is not understood, but this news about THC and serotonin may provide a clue.

CHAPTER 22

MOVEMENT DISORDERS

Movement disorders are a cluster of diseases characterized by impaired motor function and difficulties with muscle control. Basically, people who suffer from movement disorders have problems controlling how their bodies move. Their muscles and body parts may be slow to respond when their brains signal them to move, and they may have tremors, muscle spasms, lack of coordination, and sudden, spontaneous involuntary motions (not the same as seizures).

The causes of movement disorders in many cases are not well understood. Some progress is being made in finding neurological roots for these problems, involving dysfunctions or chemical imbalances in the parts of the nervous system that regulate motor motor control. Movement disorders can also arise as side effects of psychiatric medications and from impurities present in underground drugs, or as reactions to the inhalation of toxic fumes

Cannabis has proved to be helpful for some movement disorders. The reason may have to do with the presence of receptors for cannabinoids in the _basal ganglia,_ a part of the nervous system involved in the coordination of movement.

DYSTONIA

Dystonias are a group of movement disorders characterized by abnormal body movements and postures. One example of dystonia is the well-known "writer's cramp." Some cases of dystonia are _idiopathic_ meaning that their cause is unknown. Others appear to be hereditary. Dystonia can also be a side effect of medications used to treat psychotic conditions and Parkinson's disease.

CANNABIS AND DYSTONIA

Cannabis has been shown to be helpful for dystonia in studies with both humans and animals Conventional medicines used for this condition are hardly ever completely effective and can have very problematic side effects. People can use cannabis in conjunction with standard medications for a more effective overall treatment.

PARKINSON'S DISEASE

Parkinson's Disease is a movement disorder closely associated with the aging process. In fact, it has been speculated that if all of us lived long enough, we would all get Parkinson's Disease. The causes of Parkinson's Disease are thought to be abnormalities in the *basal ganglia* and the deterioration of the brain systems associated with the brain chemical *dopamine*, which is involoved in movement and motor control. Levels of dopamine decline with aging. This decline is associated with increased release of another neurotransmiter called *acetylcholine*. High levels of acetylcholine, which stimulates motor activity, have been linked to the symptoms of Parkinson's disease.

Parkinson's is sometimes called the "shaking palsy" because of the high-speed body tremors, particularly in the hands, associated with the condition. Parkinson's is also characterized by overall loss of motor control, bent posture, dystonia, and decline of sexual functioning—especially in men.

Conventional treatments for Parkinsons's disease include Deprenyl, bromocriptine, and L-dopa, all medicines which increase levels of dopamine in the nervous system. L-dopa, the most frequently used of these treatments, may actually *increase* damage to the parts of the brain involved in dopamine manufacture, and therefore does not slow down the overall progression of the disease or increase the life expectancy of those who suffer from it. Side effects of L-dopa can include nausea, vomiting, irritability, insomnia, loss of appetite, and headache. Higher dosages of L-dopa can even result in small involuntary body movements, coordination problems, hand tremors, twitching, dystonias, and muscle spasms—oddly enough, all symptoms that are very similar to those of the disease this drug is intended to treat. Bromocriptine and

Deprenyl can be used to reduce the amount of L-dopa that necessary for a Parkinson's patient to take, and therefore can also reduce the incidence and intensity of various side effects. The use of Deprenyl in Parkinson's patients actually slows down the progression of the disease and increases their life expectancy. Bromocriptine and Deprenyl generally feature fewer side effects than L-dopa.

CANNABIS AND PARKINSON'S DISEASE

Cannabis may be helpful for Parkinson's disease because it has been shown to be helfpul with other movement disorders. Some patients have used cannabis successfully to treat dystonias resulting from Parkinsons's. Furthermore, cannabis' long history of use as an aphrodisiac suggests that it might be valuable for those who suffer from the decline of sexual functioning in Parkinson's disease. Cannabidiol, one of the ingredients in cannabis, may, however, actually aggravate the *hypokinesia*, or overall lack of movement, associated with Parkinson's.

In the alleviation of the side effects of L-dopa, the main treatment for Parkinson's, cannabis might prove to be extremely helpful. As mentioned above, these side effects include nausea, vomiting, irritability, insomnia, loss of appetite, headache, dystonias, and muscle spasms. Cannabis has demonstrated a beneficial impact on them.

CHAPTER 23

MULTIPLE SCLEROSIS

Multiple sclerosis (MS) is a disease that destroys the sheathing that protects nerve fibers, thereby interfering with the function of the nervous system. As the disease progresses, the sufferer experiences painful muscle spasms, loss of coordination, tremors, paralysis, insomnia, and a wide variety of other symptoms. There are three kinds of multiple sclerosis: one which is fairly mild, and doesn't get worse over time; one which gets worse slowly; and one which gets worse very rapidly once it has appeared. Many sufferers of multiple sclerosis end up using wheelchairs.

The causes of multiple sclerosis are unkown. Scientists believe that it is an *autoimmune disorder*, in which the immune system attacks the nerve sheating in the way you would expect it to attack invaders like bacteria or viruses. Allergies are believed to operate according to a similar mechanism. Symptoms in the early stages of MS include muscle weakness, blurred vision, and numbness and tingling. In later stages the weakness increases. Tremors, problems with speaking, loss of bladder control, painful muscle spasms, mood swings and depression, and impotence can add to the victim's misery.

Modern medicine has failed to provide an effective treatment for the overall condition, although various drugs can provide short-term relief of different symptoms. Valium and similar tranquilizers, for instance, can be used to treat the muscle spasms, but these drugs frequently present problems with addiction, and the doses often have to be increased sharply over time.

Use of cannabis has been demonstrated to be helpful in treating the symptoms of multiple sclerosis. Scientific evidence suggests that cannabis helps by suppressing the action of the immune system that makes it attack the body's own cells. In animal studies , THC has been shown to protect brain cells from a kind of inflammation that accompanies an MS-like conditions. MS patients who use cannabis report that it soothes the painful muscle spasms, allowing them to limit the amount of addictive Valium-like drugs that they have to use. It can help with blurred vision, tremors, muscle coordination, and loss of bladder control, and overcomes insomnia.

For some MS victims, the use of cannabis even appears to slow down the overall progression of the disease. Patients have reported improvements such as being able to to walk unaided when they were previously unable to do so. Some have experienced a return of sexual potency. Cannabis is known to soothe mood swings and depression, and no doubt helps MS sufferers cope with these symptoms. Most multiple sclerosis patients who use cannabis find out about the benefits of the herb from support groups or word of mouth.

CHAPTER 24

NAUSEA, APPETITE LOSS, AND LOW BODY WEIGHT

Nausea and vomiting are symptomatic of many medical conditions, and can obviously result not only in loss of interest in food but in the inability to keep it down when it is consumed. Loss of appetite can be caused by nausea and vomiting, or can occur in addition to them or by itself as part of many problems and disorders. If nausea, vomiting, or loss of appetite persist for any length of time, adequate nutrition is not available to fuel the body's fight against disease, and life-threatening loss of weight can occur.

One of the most outstanding medicinal values of cannabis is the role that it can play in restoring a person's relationship to food through three channels. First, cannabis is remarkably powerful in combating nausea and vomiting, making it possible for the person to consume food and to hold it down. Secondly, it is an extraordinary stimulant of appetite itself. The third channel is the sensory enhancement and enrichment of aesthetic appreciation that cannabis so often awakens. This property expands the enjoyment of the sight, aroma, taste, and texture of food into new dimensions, transforming a simple meal into an adventure of sensation. The obsessive interest in food sometimes created by the combination of increased appetite and magnification of food's enjoyable qualities has been known for decades among social users of cannabis by the colloquial expression, "the munchies."

These properties of cannabis—reduction of nausea and vomiting, increase of appetite, and enhanced enjoyment of food—can combine to restore a healthy relationship with food in people among whom absence of appetite, loss of body weight, and inadequacy of nutrition have become dangerous and life-threatening. Conditions characterized by nausea, vomiting, appetite problems, and severe weight loss include kidney failure, tuberculosis, *hyperemesis gravidarum* which is a greatly magnified form of morning sickness and anorexia. The wasting syndrome is excessive weight loss associated with AIDS and the complications of cancer chemotherapies. These two conditions are responsible for much of the present interest in medicinal uses of cannabis.

AIDS WASTING SYNDROME

Ninety-eight percent of those with HIV, the virus generally thought to cause AIDS, experience some loss of weight. AIDS patients experience nausea and loss of appetite as the disease progresses, sometimes causing severe malnutrition and weight loss in the life-threatening "AIDS wasting syndrome." The medications standardly used to combat the HIV often cause further nausea and vomiting. Among these medicines are AZT (zidovudine) and the more recently appearing series of protease inhibitors. Added in the last few years to the arsenal of treatments for AIDS-related conditions is foscarnet or Foscavir, which unfortunately, like AZT and the protease inhibitors, also can cause severe nausea.

Antiemetic medicines that inhibit vomiting and antinauseant medicines that reduce nausea can be effective in controlling nausea in AIDS suffers, but they don't always restore lost appetite, a factor which limits their utility in treating AIDS wasting syndrome. Synthetically-produced THC (Marinol) was Federally approved in 1993 for stimulating appetite and requires a doctor's prescription.

CANNABIS AND WEIGHT GAIN

Among the arsenal of antiemetics and antinauseants available to AIDS sufferers, none approach the power of cannabis and its pharmaceutical sister, Marinol, in restoring appetite and a healthy enjoyment of food. In one study Marinol was found to relieve nausea and produce significant weight gain in seventy percent of AIDS patients.

However, approximately twenty percent of the patients found Marinol's mental effects including anxiety and disorientation so unpleasant that they ceased to use the drug. These effects are quite distinct from those of cannabis because other cannabinoids present in cannabis modulate, moderate, and augment the psychoactive effects of THC.

Another downside of Marinol is the problem of maintaining an ongoing effective level of THC in the blood for combating nausea and vomiting. Because smoking is a much more rapid and effective way of delivering THC to the bloodstream, it is easier to adjust one's dosage by smoking than by using THC in pill form, which is absorbed more slowly and less efficiently.

NAUSEA FROM CANCER CHEMOTHERAPY

Nausea and vomiting, which can last for days after a single treatment and be so violent as to threaten to break bones and rupture the esophagus, are common side effects of the chemotherapies used in treating cancer. Many patients develop such a strong aversion to the sight or odor of food that they stop eating completely and lose the will to live. Sometimes the suffering caused by chemotherapy is so great that patients choose to discontinue treatment.

Phenothiazines, which are major tranquilizers used in the treatment of severe mental illness, have been found to be effective in controlling the nausea and vomiting associated with cancer chemotherapy. Among these are Compazine, Kytril, and prochlorperazine. Zofran (ondansetron) is generally considered to be the most effective of conventional treatments. Unfortunately, Zofran, which is expensive—costing as much as six hundred dollars a treatment—must be administered by way of an intravenous drip over a period of several hours, requiring that the patient remain in a hospital bed to receive the drug.

As many as forty percent of cancer patients undergoing chemotherapy simply don't respond to standard antiemetics, drugs used to prevent vomiting. Marinol was approved for this indication in 1986 and has proven effective in many cases where other drugs failed. Similarly, smoking cannabis to control vomiting often provides relief when standard antiemetics do not help. In one study, use of cannabis was found to be effective for ninety-four percent of the bone cancer patients studied. The effectiveness of cannabis in treating nausea and vomiting from cancer chemotherapy is dose-related. The higher the blood levels of THC, the more complete the relief of vomiting. Lester Grinspoon, M.D., a psychiatrist at Harvard Medical School and co-author of *Marihuana: The Forbidden Medicine,* calculated that using cannabis to treat chemotherapy nausea would cost about one percent as much as treatment with Zofran.

A 1990 survey of about a thousand oncologists, doctors specialized in cancer treatment, indicated that they considered smoking marijuana more effective than taking Marinol and "roughly as safe." Furthermore, scientific studies have indicated that smoking is a more efficient means than oral THC of achieving high blood levels of THC, the *sine qua non* of effective relief.

Someone who is severely nauseated may have trouble keeping Marinol down long enough for it to take effect. The same problems present themselves with cannabis-containing foods. Furthermore, foods are often repulsive to people suffering from chemotherapy-induced nausea. Many patients and doctors have reported that smoking one cannabis cigarette about twenty minutes prior to a chemotherapy session—and occasionally smaller amounts after the treatment if needed—is a very effective means of controlling nausea.

RADIATION THERAPY

Like chemotherapy, radiation therapy, which many consider to be the "wave of the future" for many forms of cancer, is associated with severe nausea, markedly decreased appetite, and consequent loss of weight. Radiation therapy also causes intense pain from "radiation burn" in the area of the body radiated. Smoked cannabis has provided some patients with immense relief from all these symptoms, allowing patients to eat and return to healthy weight levels.

CHAPTER 25

SKIN CONDITIONS

Severe itching and inflamation of the skin, known as *pruritis* can be very difficult to treat. One form, called *contact dermatitis* results from exposure of the skin to an allergen, irritant, or toxin. The offending substances can include household and workplace chemicals like acids, solvents, and cleansers—anything that dries out the skin by removing the protective layer of fat. The most common irritants that cause contact dermatitis are detergents and simple hot water. Besides itching, symptoms include red, cracked, and oozing areas of skin. Contact dermatitis usually passes when exposure to the irritant is discontinued.

Atopic dermatitis another form of chronic skin condition whose cause is suspected to be related to a deficiency in immune function. The condition also appears to be related to stress, and often becomes more severe during stressful periods. Symptoms of atopic dermatitis are itching rash particularly in areas where the skin retains moisture and heat, such as the skin creases of the elbows, knees, neck, face, hands, feet, genital areas, and buttocks. The skin becomes dry and thickened in these areas. The severity of the itching can cause ongoing insomnia, resulting chronic tiredness. Scratching can become compulsive, unconscious, and out of the person's control, resulting in breaking of skin, infection, and scarring. People with atopic dermatitis may be more vulnerable to fungal and viral infections and to adverse reactions to drugs and vaccinations.

People at high risk for atopic dermatitis are those who have hay fever, asthma, or food allergies and those who have a family history of atopic dermatitis. People who use drugs that interfere with the functioning of the immune system seem to be at high risk for atopic dermatitis.

CONVENTIONAL TREATMENTS

Dermatitis is usually treated with corticosteroids and ointments applied to the skin. However, corticosteroids can only be used safely for brief acute periods because long-term use usually entails severe side effects. Antihistamines can be used to control pruritis, but their effectiveness in this regard is usually limited. Sedatives and tranquilizers are sometimes used in more severe dermatitis because of the various ways that the condition is related to stress. These drugs can help moderate the stress that triggers increased severity of the condition, as well as the stress and tension caused by constant itching and the complications that can result, such as infections and disfigurement of the skin. Such drugs can also help permit sleep when itching and pain are intense enough to interfere with it. Unfortunately, these drugs are highly addictive and feature rapid development of tolerance. Antibiotics are used to treat the infections resulting from uncontrolled scratching. Unfortunately, even all of these treatments taken together constitute very limited help for people suffering from severe dermatitis.

CANNABIS AND DERMATITIS

Although it no doubt comes as a surprise to most people who haven't had or been exposed to a severe case of dermatitis, this perplexing condition can be personally, socially, and professionally debilitating—even life life-threatening. And consequently, cannabis, which is sometimes dramatically more effective than conventional treatments, can therefore be a life-renewing treatment.

Nineteenth-century doctors noticed cannabis' efficacy in anaesthetizing the skin, relieving itching, and permitting sleep. Historical accounts describe one such medical practitioner who treated a case of triple addiction—to alcohol and injections of morphine and cocaine—that resulted from another doctor's efforts to self-medicate a severe skin problem.

ONE MAN'S MISERY

In 1987 hearings before the Drug Enforcement Agency (DEA) regarding the legal status of cannabis, one man suffering from atopic dermatitis provided testimony that demonstrated the tragic potential of the condition, the inadequacy of conventional treatments, and the outstanding benefits that cannabis can offer some sufferers. He described how, when he was young, his hands and arms were so shredded from splitting of the skin and scratching that they had become infected with gangrene. The situation was serious enough to be life-threatening, so doctors asked his parents' permission to amputate both of his arms at the elbow—although they did not ultimately carry through with this course of action. For the years that followed, his skin disfigurement was so horrendous that he had trouble getting work simply because of how he looked. And when he did get employment, he had to take so much time off for his condition that we was dismissed. He lost his marriage and became socially withdrawn. A full, ongoing battery of conventional treatments, including Valium, Librium, and cortisone—which after a time he could no longer use because of concern about adverse effects—provided no long-term relief.

This man's misery persisted until he took his first few puffs of a cannabis cigarette, offered to him socially by a man who was at that time just about his only friend. This small dose, to his amazement, made the itching that had plagued him every day for many years go away completely for several days! After the itching came back, it disappeared again with only one puff. Subsequent experimentation proved that a total of two to three cannabis cigarettes, on weekends only, kept the dermatitis sufficiently under control that it presented *no symptoms at all* unless he interrupted this very light regimen of cannabis use. (Oddly enough, this man testified that he never noticed *any* psychoactive effect). He was able to get and hold a job and begin to lead a much more fulfilling life.

The mechanism by which cannabis can quickly and completely clear up a long-term case of atopic dermatitis, as in this case, simply isn't known. Cases such as this one suggest the possibility that cannabis may make a biological intervention in the confusing underlying disease process of atopic dermatitis. If, as is suspected, atopic dermatitis stems from dysfunction of immunity, it's possible that this route of action lies in the modulation of autoimmune response that has been observed with cannabis and is suspected to play a role in its benefits to arthritic conditions.

PALLIATIVE ROUTES

However, there are a number of routes by which known palliative properties of cannabis can provide soothing help for dermatitis. First is its anti-inflammatory action. Aside from all of its potential symptoms and complications, dermatitis is an inflammation of the skin. Second are the analgesic or painkilling properties of cannabis. These may anesthetize the skin to some degree, and are no doubt at least partially responsible for the decrease in the sensation of itching that use of cannabis can bring. The anti-inflammatory and analgesic benefits can be brought about by smoking or ingesting food or tincture preparations, but cannabis could be additionally helpful in cases of dermatitis made into a poultice and applied directly to the affected areas of skin. Further value could be derived from topical application by way of the anti-infection action of cannabis, which could help with cases where skin has become infected from splitting or breaking and scratching.

The analgesic and anti-inflammatory aspects are a palliative action of cannabis that provide symptomatic relief allowing sleep where symptoms have been severe enough to interfere. Here, these actions supplement the sleep-inducing, sedative properties of cannabis to encourage deep and restful sleep and consequently relieve chronic tiredness from the insomnia that sometimes complicates dermatitis.

Quite remarkably, these palliative actions of cannabis, in situations where it works well for dermatitis, fold into a single medication virtually all of the functions of the diverse conventional treatments that otherwise must be used to treat dermatitis. Cannabis, both ingested and applied topically, performs the anti-inflammatory and pruritis-reducing roles of corticosteroids that are administered topically and taken internally, as well as accomplishing the relief of itching sought in the ingestion of antihistamines. Cannabis in topical form also duplicates or augments the antibiotic function of other medicines that are part of the conventional armamentarium of treatments for the complications of dermatitis, and acts in the sleep-inducing capacity of the tranquilizers that are sometimes also prescribed.

The entire range and diversity of cannabis' beneficial palliative functions for chronic dermatitis, however, fail to encompass what may be the most valuable property of cannabis for this condition: its psychoactive action. Atopic dermatitis is connected to stress, and it has been shown that the severity of the condition often increases with raised stress levels. If stress is indeed at the core of this condition, the role of this trigger would help to explain its chronic nature, for this disturbing, perplexing, and recalcitrant condition itself *causes* a great deal of stress, a factor which would tend to keep the entire disease process in motion. The stress-reducing capacity of cannabis—which is part of its psychoactive property—may interrupt this stress cycle more effectively with less risk of addiction than conventional tranquilizers and sedatives for many patients. Indeed, several doctors have recognized the centrality of the euphoriant and relaxant effects in providing relief for dermatitis-type problems.

Some doctors believe that skin conditions, along with the related disorders of allergies and asthma are often of *psychosomatic* origin, meaning that the cause of the symptoms lies in the patient's mental state. This viewpoint goes further than the observation that stress aggravates these conditions to say that mental factors are responsible for the appearance of the disorder in the first place. To whatever extent this is the case, such a mental component in the disease would open a window through which a beneficial, positive psychoactive effect, such as that uniquely provided by cannabis, could offer assistance. Perhaps the psychoactivity of cannabis, in particular the relaxation response that it elicits, may well be the key to its benefits in skin disorders.

Looking at the combination of palliative and psychoactive benefits in the use of cannabis for skin disorders highlights the therapeutic importance of the combined action of the beneficial cannabinoids naturally present in the plant. Those cannabinoids, such as CBD, most closely associated with analgesic, anti-inflammatory, and sedative action—palliative benefits for skin disorders—are not the same as those mostly connected with the herb's positive psychoactivity, which include the various forms of THC. Thus, the overall, holistic benefit provided by cannabis could not be duplicated by isolated pharmaceutical versions of individual components.

CHAPTER 26

WITHDRAWAL FROM DRUG ADDICTION

*O*piates are a class of powerful sedative painkilling drugs derived from a beautiful flowering plant called the *opium poppy*. Opium is an extract prepared from the plant with a long history of use in the Middle and Far East. Morphine is another powerful opiate that gained widespread use in Western medicine in the nineteenth century and is still an important painkilling tool today. Heroin, a more potent chemical deriviative of morphine, was developed as a substitute for morphine during withdrawal and is no longer used by doctors. Heroin is the basis of a huge international underground black market.

Opiates are highly addictive, physically and psychologically, entrapping the user in a vise-like grip. Another surge of black market opiate use, especially heroin, began in the 1990s among all ethnic, social, and economic groups, ensnaring professional and educated as well as impoverished and socially marginalized people.

The addictive power of opiates springs from their relationship to endorphins, the body's natural neurochemicals responsible for controlling pain and producing pleasure. Opiates mimic the action of endorphins and interact with the same receptor sites in the human nervous system that are used by endorphins. In habitual opiate use, opiates quickly usurp the function of the body's natural endorphins, causing the body to reduce production of these native pain-controlling, "feel-good" neurochemicals. Thus, when opiate use is suddenly discontinued, neither normal levels of endorphins nor their opiate imitators are available to hold pain in check and provide feelings of pleasure. It takes the body a while to restore endorphin production to natural levels. In the meantime, the deficiency of endorphins produces the syndrome of intense suffering known as withdrawal. The urgency of avoiding this condition is the most powerful fuel driving the engine of heroin addiction.

Opiate withdrawal is a nightmare. The apt street term for this condition is "dopesickness." The syndrome, which can be quite pronounced even if heroin has been used steadily for only three days or more, is characterized by agitation, feverishness, insomnia, irritability, mood swings, sweating, nausea, vomiting, increased mucus production which creates symptoms resembling those of a head cold, diarrhea, generalized body pain, muscle soreness, overstimulation, mental confusion, and in more severe cases, tremors and muscle spasms.

The singularly hellish nature of opiate withdrawal, however, can't be fully understood in terms of its symptoms. There is an additional quality that combines with whatever symptoms are experienced to make dopesickness so undesirable as to compel entrenched opiate habitués to avoid it—sometimes even at the cost of a lifetime disruptive, taxing, expensive, and socially stigmatizing drug habit. This is a psychological factor, a cloud of mental despair that pervades the withdrawal experience. The cause of this feeling is probably the low levels of endorphin activity during this transitional period. In addition to performing various physiological functions and regulating the amount of pain we experience, endorphins also play crucial roles in mental state, producing feelings of general well-being. This is why surges of endorphin activity, like those experienced during certain kinds of exercise, make us feel so good. The relative absence of this function of endorphins during opiate withdrawal is the biochemical root of the ubiquitous undertone of emotional and mental desperation permeating withdrawal.

Withdrawal symptoms usually peak on the third consecutive day that opiates have not been used, abating rapidly thereafter. During the first three or four days of withdrawal the sufferer will probably need tranquilizers or sleep medicine. It is reported to last an eternity. When an opiate habit is maintained for a long period, the dosage regularly used tends to increase due to tolerance. Both of these factors—the duration of the habit and the size of the dose—influence the nature of withdrawal. The longer the habit has lasted and the higher the regular dose, the worse the withdrawal will be, entrenching ever more deeply the motivation to perpetuate the habit, and decreasing the chances of kicking it successfully.

TREATMENTS FOR OPIATE ADDICTION AND WITHDRAWAL

A highly addictive synthetic opiate called methadone is the most common conventional approach to treating heroin addiction and withdrawal. Methadone is a pharmeceutical substitute for heroin prescribed to prevent withdrawal symptoms when heroin use is discontinued. Addicts accepted into a methadone program visit a clinic every day, where they are administered on site a controlled quantity of the drug in drink form. Methadone programs provide addicts with a structured, predictable, relatively safe alternative to the chaos, stress, financial expense, and legal and health risks that can be part of dependence on the black market heroin trade. Patients can be placed on a program of methadone "maintenance," in which the same dose of methadone will be provided everyday for an indefinite period. Alternatively, or after such a maintenance period, the dose of methadone can be slowly reduced in a controlled fashion that minimizes withdrawal symptoms.

Unfortunately, there are many problems with methadone programs, although they work well for many individuals. Methadone is *more* physically addictive than heroin, and is therefore not a cure for addiction but a form of "harm reduction". Some patients find the side effects of methadone, like severe sedation and bloating, to be worse than those of heroin. They may complicate their problems by using other problematic drugs, like speed, to counteract the sedation. Additionally, methadone doesn't provide the kind of psychoactive high that makes heroin attractive. Many addicts supplement the prescription methadone with street heroin, creating an addiction even more complex than that which compelled them to seek treatment.

A growing range of other treatments and drug-substitution therapies for heroin addiction are becoming available through the medical establishment. A cocktail of tranquilizers and painkillers, or "kick kit," is often prescribed on a short term basis to soothe withdrawal symptoms, although most patients who use this approach find that withdrawal is still excruciating. In spite of the diverse options available, the prognosis for recovery without relapse from chronic opiate addiction remains discouraging no matter which approach is used.

CANNABIS AND OPIATE ADDICTION

Cannabis has a substantial track record as a remarkably effective palliative for the discomfort that persists for several days after stopping regular opiate use. Doctors in the nineteenth century frequently used cannabis tinctures for this purpose. One American doctor from this period, J. B. Mattison, M.D., devoted his career to the treatment of addiction, or "narcotic inebriety," as the condition was then called. He extensively documented the power of cannabis tinctures in treating addictions to morphine and opium poppy extract, a problem that was widespread in the United States in the end of the nineteenth century. Although some cases responded more fully than others, sometimes cannabis, without any other painkillers, was all that was required to get a person through the withdrawal period and thence free from the opiate. One such case from Mattison's records has made medical history, that of a naval surgeon who had been injecting large doses of morphine every day for nine years. Less than a dozen doses of cannabis extract were required to complete successful treatment in this instance of severe, chronic opiate dependency.

A controlled study of the use of THC in the treatment of opiate dependency was conducted in the twentieth century under the auspices of Mayor Fiorello LaGuardia of New York City, who appointed a special commission to study it. Withdrawal symptoms among a sizable group given THC were compared to those of a control group. The THC was found to be useful in diminishing, and in some cases even completely eliminating, the discomfort of heroin withdrawal. Additonally, withdrawal symptoms tended to be of shorter duration. The initial inspiration to conduct this research came from an observation that the psychoactive high produced by cannabis was sufficiently similar to that produced by the opiates to suggest the possibility that it might be valuable in treating opiate withdrawal.

The *North Carolina Journal of Medicine*, 1953 edition, reported success in the use of parahexyl, an artificial cannabinoid made by modifying the chemical structure of natural cannabinoids to increase potency, for treating the symptoms of withdrawal from opiates and alcohol. Since then, little if any research in this area has been conducted, and no contemporary conventional treatment of opiate addiction includes the use of cannabis. The tradition of using cannabis for opiate withdrawal continues today among underground of users of black market opiates, some of whom are aware of cannabis' helpful properties. Many of them have found that eating very potent cannabis food preparations is much more effective for withdrawal than is smoking. Some may continue to use cannabis after the withdrawal period is over, finding that it helps soften the *psychological* craving for opiates that may still arise and compels many abstaining heroin users to fall off the wagon. They say that the soothing high offered by cannabis fills the void left by opiates, without the dangers of street opiates. In some cases cannabis may be appropriate as a long-term substitute for opiate use.

Cannabis' value in treating opiate withdrawal and in serving as a harm-reducing substitute for opiates derives from its palliative and psychoactive effects. As a palliative, cannabis' painkilling properties soothe the body pains, muscle soreness, and hypersensitivity to pain that characterize withdrawal. The sedative effects take the edge off the agitation and hyperstimulation suffered during withdrawal, and facilitate sleep. Cannabis also functions as an antipyretic, or fever-reducing substance, thus ameliorating the feverishness, chills, and sweating that can occur during dopesickness. It also relieves nausea and vomiting, and restores lost appetite. In the experiments conducted under Mayor LaGuardia, THC relieved the diarrhea that accompanied heroin withdrawal.

The LaGuardia experiments revealed a factor that had been largely overlooked in the literature on medicinal use of cannabis and its derivatives. Dr. Roger Adam's report on this study states that "the feeling of euphoria...helped in rehabilitating the physical condition and in facilitating social reorientation. An outstanding result is a subjective feeling of relaxation."

Although the variety of palliative effects of cannabis that help in opiate withdrawal are quite remarkable, it can be argued that cannabis' psychoactivity may well be its most crucial asset for facilitating an effective transition out of opiate use. The despair and hopelessness characterizing the withdrawal period are not addressed by the tranquilizers and pain medications usually prescribed to relieve symptoms. The mental negativity, despair, and hopelessness of withdrawal often sabotage attempts to kick opiates by permeating the thoughts and beliefs the patient formulates about being able to go through the withdrawal period and subsequent abstinence. The mental darkness of withdrawal creates an expectation of failure, and with this anticipation the effort to continue enduring the suffering of this time period seems futile. This negativity often generates a self-fulfilling prophecy. It is easy to see how a patient who is thinking this way is likely to give up and return to opiate use.

Cannabis' psychoactive properties have an uplifting effect. After smoking cannabis, people feel more hopeful, have more faith, are more optimistic, and express greater openness to possibility. These factors act to counter the negativity of withdrawal, making it more endurable, and thereby increasing the chances that the patient will be able to muster the necessary persistence to see the process through. Furthermore, the cannabis high has enough kinship with the psychoactivity of opiates to help reduce the patient's craving for this psychological effect of opiates. Additionally, and crucially, the optimism engendered by cannabis helps the person to have faith and hope, to *believe* that withdrawal will be successful because he or she can endure withdrawal and maintain abstinence thereafter, and that to do so will be fulfilling and rewarding. These positive expectations encourage the patient to believe that whatever suffering they may be experiencing is worthwhile, and therefore decrease the likelihood that the patient will resume opiate use before the process has been completed.

Cannabis closely mirrors much of the spectrum of the poppy's positive pain-relieving properties and desirable psychoactive effects, while possessing none of its darker powers. Furthermore, the match between the palliative properties of cannabis and the diverse vicissitudes of opiate withdrawal is also quite remarkable. Cannabis addresses to some degree virtually every symptom of opiate withdrawal. On top of this, cannabis provides a form of psychoactive assistance and encouragement well-suited to help the patient see the gloomy process of opiate withdrawal through to its end. By complementing the presence of the powerful poppy plant with the potent but gentle cannabis, it almost seems as if Nature herself has wisely and thoughtfully balanced the cornucopia of plant forms so generously offered to humankind for medicinal use.

ALCOHOL ADDICTION

Another drug for which cannabis can ease the pain of withdrawal, and for which cannabis can serve as an effective substitute, is the most widely used social drug in the United States—alcohol. Symptoms of alcohol withdrawal are somewhat similar to those of the opiates: anxiety, restlessness, insomnia, and various kinds of physical discomfort, all of which are areas where cannabis can provide relief. More severe instances of alcohol withdrawal can precipitate the syndrome known *delirium tremens*, or "D.T.'s", a fever-like condition characterized by hallucinations and mental confusion, sweating, rapid heartbeat, and muscle tremors. Nineteenth century doctors often specifically indicated cannabis for this condition, and twentieth century scientific studies have shown favorable results in the use of cannabis and cannabinoids in ameliorating the symptoms of alcohol withdrawal.

Two of the primary forces driving many cases of alcohol abuse are anxiety and depression. In fact, many doctors consider anxiety reduction to be the specific cause of a particular type of pattern of episodic drinking. Unfortunately, alcohol tends in the long-term to aggravate the anxiety and depression that many people use it to medicate. Hangovers, after all, are very depressing; and alcoholism itself, along with the complications and problems it introduces into a person's life, can in itself be a source of depression and anxiety.

Cannabis can be used not only to ease the anxiety and depression that accompany periods of withdrawal from alcohol, but can also serve as an effective substitute for alcohol by medicating the depression and anxiety that motivate many alcohol habits to begin with.

Those who have used cannabis to fill the role that alcohol once played in their lives have found that they can lead much more functional, healthy lives by smoking a joint in place of drink. Psychiatrist Tod Mikuriya, M.D., describes one such case of a woman whose therapy for a thirty-five year history of alcohol abuse began with a program of using cannabis instead whenever she felt the urge to drink. Her first discovery was that she could regulate and limit her use of cannabis so as not to interfere with routine tasks and daily functioning. Although she had often tried, she had never been able to exercise any such control over her alcohol intake which often had been totally out of control. For instance, she might get drunk and alienate friends by coming on sexually to someone else's husband at a party; or she'd walk into a bar, pick a strange man, and end up in a threatening situation; and sometimes she'd black out and wake up not knowing where she was. She found that cannabis, on the other hand, triggered no such self-destructive episodes. In describing how her life had changed since switching to cannabis, she said that she felt good, was relaxed, no longer belligerent and depressed nor bothered by trivialities whose irritation was enormously magnified under the influence of alcohol.

People have also reported that cannabis has helped them recover physically from the harsh toll exacted on their bodies from long periods of alcohol abuse.

WITHDRAWAL FROM OTHER DRUGS

Cannabis also proves helpful as a medicine for the symptoms of withdrawal from various additional addictive drugs. In the nineteenth century the herb was used to treat withdrawal from "chloral," a strong sleep-inducing barbiturate. This usage of cannabis suggests that the herb might be helpful in treating withdrawal from the tranquilizers and barbiturates used more commonly today, such as Valium and phenobarbital.

Another nineteenth century use of cannabis was the medication of withdrawal from cocaine. Both cocaine abuse and addiction to amphetamines—stimulants which have many properties in common with cocaine—is widespread in the United States today. Street users of these drugs often employ cannabis to ease the discomforts of withdrawal from these drugs when trying to kick their habits or during periods when the stimulants they normally use are unavailable.

One of the foremost characteristics of withdrawal from stimulants is depression. These substances exert a short-term antidepressive effect by increasing the levels of brain chemicals that elevate mood. However, the use of these drugs actually depletes available levels of these neurochemicals, leading to the lethargy and depression or "crash" that occur upon "coming down" from their effects. The desire to escape this depressive after-effect often inspires further use of these stimulants, initiating the mounting pattern of use that spirals into addiction. The anti-depressive, mood-elevating properties of cannabis canassist in combating the depression characteristic of the crash, helping to curb the craving for another "hit" of stimulant drugs.

Another factor that fuels stimulant addiction is the lethargy that follows discontinuation of use. People become dependent on the energy provided by stimulants to be able to accomplish tasks and get things done, much as a vast percentage of Americans rely on caffeine. People experiencing the listlessness characteristic of withdrawal from stimulants may feel incapable of getting anything done, thus motivating a return to stimulant use. The stimulant properties of THC may be of assistance here, helping those in withdrawal from drugs such as cocaine and amphetamines maintain a somewhat higher level of energy.

BENEFICIAL PALLATIVE

Cannabis turns out to be an effective medicine for withdrawal from a very broad spectrum of addictive drugs. While it can be used in conjunction with other withdrawal medications, it is sometimes sufficient by itself. The palliative and psychoactive properties both play important roles in the relief it provides for these conditions. It can even intervene biologically with withdrawal symptoms, by helping to prevent the muscle spasms and tremors of more severe opiate and alcohol withdrawal syndromes.

Cannabis can also serve as a form of "substitution therapy," providing a replacement for various addictive drugs according to the harm reduction paradigm of drug treatment. In this capacity, cannabis features the advantage of being almost entirely non-addictive. Although the use of the herb can be habit-forming in the sense of almost any substance or activity, the discontinuation of cannabis use does not carry the threat of withdrawal syndromes and severe cravings (unlike, for instance, methadone, which is even more addictive than the heroin which it is used to replace). Furthermore, the use of cannabis permits a functional, productive lifestyle among many users who could not control their behavior and fulfill their responsibilities while under the sway of alcoholism or drug addiction. Cannabis is not associated with liver damage or the other forms of physical deterioration attendant to prolonged alcohol consumption, and unlike opiates, alcohol, and tranquilizers, a fatal or coma-inducing overdose of cannabis is not possible.

LISTENING TO CANNABIS

*H*umankind's relationship to cannabis has already been long, varied, and productive. Its greatest benefits, however, are yet to unfold. The rate of discovery in our understanding of this beneficial plant is entering an exciting period of acceleration that promises to yield many fruits. Just as the bonds between human individuals grow, change, develop, and pass through distinctly different stages, the human relationship to the cannabis plant is about to blossom into a dynamic new maturity.

LISTENING TO A PLANT TEACHER

Tribes and cultures that have used cannabis and other plants for spiritual and healing purposes have long understood the principle of relating to plants as teachers. Some peoples have claimed that the cannabis high opens an inner door through which the voices of spirits can be heard, offering wisdom from the spiritual realm. Some traditions have held that the plant is itself the earthly embodiment or emissary of a powerful angelic entity that makes its voice audible to those who consume it with proper reverence for its sacred essence. These entheogenic phenomena require *listening* to the voice of the plant, as one would to the voice of a teacher, to avail oneself of the information it imparts.

A substance as widely used as cannabis is well worth listening to, for the very power and breadth of its attraction within our society indicates that it has much to tell us about ourselves. In the best-selling book, *Listening to Prozac*, a modern psychiatrist updates the ancient notion of listening to psychoactive substances, suggesting that today's most widely used pharmaceutical psychoactive may be able to help us answer fundamental questions about the biological roots of personality.

Turning such a receptive ear towards the messages of cannabis is the key to reaping maximum benefits from our relationship to this plant ally in the future. As the ears of science and medicine become increasingly attentive to the healing magic of cannabis and the revelations encoded within the plant, we will learn a great deal about our bodies, minds, and spirits, about nature and the plant world, and about the possibilities of synergy between plants and people. And a plant that heals in so many ways no doubt has valuable lessons to teach us about the nature of healing itself. As we listen to cannabis and observe the ways that it heals through biological intervention, we will learn new information about the bodily processes of disease and health. By listening to the psychoactivity of cannabis, we will gain new insight into the nature of the mind, its relationship to the body, and how states of mind change our bodily reality and shape our physiological future. By acting as an entheogen, cannabis will teach us about the mystery of faith and offer us further glimpses of our divine essence.

A CHRISTMAS STOCKING FROM NATURE

A truly remarkable aspect of cannabis' healing magic is that the plant contains over sixty medicinally active ingredients which interact and synergize. THC, for instance, is responsible for some of cannabis' stimulating and psychoactive properties, whereas CBD appears to have a more sedative action and to soften the psychoactivity of THC.

Medical research has already started to explore the medicinal properties of THC in isolation. As research into cannabis continues, the medicinal effects of different cannabinoids, and the synergies between them, will be increasingly understood. Specific cannabinoids will prove to have special value for certain conditions, whereas they or other cannabinoids may even turn out to be be undesirable in certain situations.

So far, THC in isolation has generally proven to be of less medicinal value than whole cannabis. With ongoing research, however, various cannabinoids in isolation, and even specific clusters of cannabinoids— some of them perhaps administered in higher doses than are available naturally—may prove to have extraordinary medical utility for individuals with specific conditions.

Custom-designed and balanced combinations of cannabinoids in pharmaceutical form will become available. People with special needs will be prescribed cannabinoids in dosages and proportions ideally appropriate to their conditions and proclivities. For instance, those seeking maximum painkilling effects with a minimum of psychoactivity will be able to use pharmaceutical preparations of cannabinoids whose balance of contents achieve this goal.

The practice of administering cannabinoids in this fashion will not replace the practice of using whole cannabis, which will continue to be the most valuable method for many people, but will instead come to coexist alongside it. Efforts are already underway to breed strains of cannabis especially suited to specific needs and conditions. Analysis of the cannabinoid content of strains particularly successful for specific conditions will provide clues for those researching the medicinal effects of isolated pharmaceutical cannabinoids, just as research in this area will assist in the breeding of special strains for medicinal purposes.

The art and science of cannabis-based medicine will become increasingly refined and powerful. It will become ever more apparent that cannabis is not just *one* medicine, but many, *many* medicines, of value for a widening spectrum of conditions. Our awe and reverence for Nature's wisdom and generosity in bestowing the healing gift of cannabis upon humankind will grow with each discovery about the cannabinoids, just as a child thrills anew upon discovering each separate gift hidden in a Christmas stocking packed to the brim with wonder after wonder.

BOON FOR SENIORS

The medicinal benefits of cannabis are especially suited to the elderly. Arthritis, depression, movement disorders, sleep problems, and chronic pain, for instance, conditions prevalent among elderly people, and are all conditions for which cannabis has medicinal value. Cannabis is most widely recognized for its utility in soothing the nausea and vomiting associated with chemotherapies, and cancer also occurs with higher incidence among the elderly. As the baby boom generation reaches maturity the size of the elderly population will grow to an unprecedented level. Because cannabis is so well-suited to conditions that accompany aging, its importance will expand dramatically with this demographic shift.

In the decade to come, those who came of age during the turbulent decade of the 1960s—the crest of the baby boom—will be reaching retirement age. This more than any previous generation is favorably disposed towards cannabis because the massive leap in its use that began the 1960s was initiated by them. Furthermore, the entrance of this generation into its elderly years coincides with an explosion of public interest in cannabis' medicinal properties.

These factors will combine to generate a far greater use of cannabis among the elderly than previously anticipated. Medicinal cannabis will become a major boon to the aging in America. Huge numbers of aging people will prefer to avoid the toxic and debilitating effects of the multiple pharmaceuticals often prescribed for conditions of aging and will turn to a beneficial plant of whose safety they have been assured by personal experience.

As baby boomers discover cannabis' extraordinary medicinal efficacy for elderly people, many will feel that the greatest benefits of cannabis are wasted on the young. The traditional association of cannabis with youth may, in fact, become reversed as it comes to be thought of as a palliative ally especially suited to the senior years.

USE OR ABUSE?

As the healing properties of cannabis—formerly dismissed by our society as a "drug of abuse"—become more apparent to greater numbers of people, it will also become clearer that the motivation underlying much of the use and abuse of "recreational" or illegal drugs is medicinal—reflecting a search for healing on some level of body, mind, or spirit. Instead of waging war on those whose desperate gropings towards healing have led them into the tangle of a drug problem, society may instead attempt to help them achieve the healing that they seek. Such efforts will be assisted by the recognition that in many cases cannabis can actually serve as an effective agent in helping break free of drug abuse.

By relegating cannabis to the status of a dangerous drug of abuse, or accepting the caricature of cannabis as a relatively harmless drug that nonetheless makes people slow and stupid, society perpetrates a form of "drug abuse" quite different from that normally implied by the phrase. For in not acknowledging and respecting cannabis' extraordinary value, society abuses cannabis in the same sense that we would abuse a grand piano if we used it only as a doorstop. In condemning cannabis, or in using it with casual, mindless disregard for the healing opportunities it presents, we fail to *listen* to the voice of the plant. In this failing, we as a society abuse cannabis just as we as individuals abuse our loved ones when we don't listen to their urgently uttered words. And in this failing we abuse *ourselves* by not availing our ears of cannabis' healing music.

Drug abuse, after all, arises from *not listening*. It comes from not listening to the potentially medicinal substances around us and what they have to tell us about their powers and possibilities, positive and negative. It comes from not listening to our bodies and how they react to the substances we put inside them. It comes from not listening to our minds, the wise judgments of informed intellect and the cautious counsel of reason. It comes from not listening to our spirits and instead dampening the soul's cry for healing by medicating ourselves into deafness. And it comes from not listening to those who care about us.

Those concerned about abusing cannabis, then, are well advised to listen. By listening closely to the voice of the plant as it can be heard through body, mind, and spirit, you will be able to discern whether you are abusing cannabis or making healing use of it. Listen to your body. Is your use of cannabis achieving the painkilling or soothing effects that you desire? Or are you using so much cannabis that your body is not enlivened but numbed, its voice silenced? Listen to your mind. Are you achieving optimism, constructive detachment and creative thinking, or are you using so much cannabis that your mind is dulled, prompting you not to *re*-consider but rather not to consider at all? And listen to your spirit, to what the Quakers called the "still, small voice within." Can you hear it? Does your use of cannabis seem to amplify or to dull the voice of the inner self?

Listen as well to your doctor, health practitioners, caretakers, and loved ones about what they have observed concerning your use of cannabis and its effects. Listening and responding to honest and thoughtful feedback is one of the best means of avoiding drug abuse. Fortunately, cannabis is kind and forgiving, and even if over-used or "abused" it has minimal ill effects.

CANNABIS PROMOTES LISTENING

Fortunately as well, cannabis promotes listening itself. By amplifying subtle physiological sensations, cannabis helps us to listen to our bodies, recognize and release physical tension, and pay heed to signs of stress and disease as well as signs of healing. By amplifying the senses, cannabis compels us to listen to the voice of beauty in all that surrounds us. By promoting humor and laughter, cannabis helps us to listen to and to *get* the healing cosmic joke. By promoting conviviality and social engagement, cannabis encourages us to listen to *each other*. By affording a detached perspective that allows us to observe our feelings and thought processes, cannabis helps us to listen to our minds and to dispute our thoughts when they have become poisoned with pessimism and clogged with gloom. By acting as an entheogen, cannabis helps us to listen to the spirit of faith and hope within ourselves, the inner voice that stirs the body's healing energies.

Let us open our ears, listen to the song of cannabis, and thank Nature for this healing gift.

REFERENCES

Abel, E. L., Marihuana: The First Twelve Thousand Years, Plenum, 1980.

Adams, Roger, "Marijuana," Bulletin New York Academy of Medicine, 18 (1942), reprinted in Marijuana: Medical Papers edited by Tod. H. Mikuriya.

Allentuck, S., and K. M. Bowman, "The Psychiatric Aspects of Marihuana Intoxication," American Journal of Psychiatry 99 (1942).

Amentano, Paul, "Australian Government Takes Objective Look at Medical Marijuana," High Times, January 1996.

Anonymous, "Prayer to Saint Joseph," The Regina Press, (prayer card).

Bello, Joan, The Benefits of Marijuana: Physical, Psychological, and Spiritual, Sweetlight Books, 1996.

Bennett, Chris, Lynn Osburn, and Judy Osburn, Green Gold, The Tree of Life: Marijuana in Magic and Religion, Access Unlimited, 1995.

Benson, Herbert, with Marg Stark, "Reason to Believe," Natural Health, May-June 1996.

Benson, Herbert, with Marg Stark, Timeless Healing: The Power and Biology of Belief, Scribner, 1996.

Birch, E. A., "The Use of Indian Hemp in the Treatment of Chronic Chloral and Chronic Opium Poisoning," Lancet 1 (1889).

Boire, Richard Glen, Marijuana Law, 2nd Edition, Ronin Publishing, 1996.

Braude, M. C., and S. Szara, eds., Pharmacology of Marihuana (2 v.), Raven Press, 1976.

Burgess, G. Anthony, Indoor Sinsemilla, G., 1984.

Carver, G. W., How to Grow Marijuana Indoors for Medicinal Use, Sun Magic Publishing, 1997.

Cervantes, Jorge, Robert Connell Clarke, and Ed Rosenthal, Indoor Marijuana Horticulture, Revised, 1993.

Cherniak, Laurence, The Great Books of Hashish: Volume I, Book I: Morocco, Lebanon, Afghanistan, the Himalayas, And/Or, 1979.

Cherniak, Laurence, The Great Books of Hashish: Volume I, Book II: Marijuana Around The World, Sinsemilla, Stash, Opium, Cherniak/Damele Publishing Co., 1982.

Clarke, Robert Connell, Marijuana Botany: The Propagation and Breeding of Distinctive Cannabis, Ronin Publishing, 1981.

Clifford, D. B., "Tetrahydrocannabinol for Tremor in Multiple Sclerosis," Annals of Neurology 13 (1983).

Cohen, Jessica, "The Greatest Story Never Told," Utne Reader, April 1997.

Cohen, Sidney, and Richard Stillman, eds., The Therapeutic Potential of Marijuana, Plenum, 1975.

Cone, Tracie, "Reefer Madness," San Jose Mercury News, May 14, 1995.

Conrad, Chris, Hemp for Health: The Medicinal and Nutritional Uses of Cannabis Sativa, Healing Arts Press, 1997.

Conrad, Chris, Hemp: Lifeline to the Future, Creative Xpressions, 1993.

Consroe, P. F., G. C. Wood, and H. Buchsbaum, "Anticonvulsant Nature of Marihuana Smoking," Journal of the American Medical Association 234 (1975).

Consroe, P., R. Sandyk, and S. R. Snider, "Open Label Evaluation of Cannabidiol in Dystonic Movement Disorders," International Journal of Neuroscience 30 (1982).

Cousins, Norman, Head First: The Biology of Hope, E. P. Dutton, 1989.

Cunha, J. M., E. A. Carlini, A. E. Pereira, et al., "Chronic Administration of Cannabidiol to Healthy Volunteers and Epileptic Patients," Pharmacology 21 (1980).

Devereaux, Paul, The Long Trip: A Prehistory of Psychedelia, Arkana, 1997.

Diamond, W. John, W. Lee Cowden, and Burton Goldberg, An Alternative Medicine Definitive Guide to Cancer, Future Medicine Publishing, Inc., 1997.

Dilman, Vladimir M., and Ward Dean, The Neuroendocrine Theory of Aging and Degenerative Disease, The Center for Bio-Gerontology, 1992.

Doblin, R., and M. A. R. Kleinman, "Marihuana as Anti-emetic Medicine: A Survey of Oncologists' Attitudes and Experiences," Journal of Clinical Oncology 9 (1991).

Doblin, Rick, "Marijuana and AIDS Wasting Syndrome Protocol," MAPS, Spring 1996.

Drake, Bill, Marijuana: The Cultivator's Handbook, Ronin Publishing, Inc., 1986.

Drake, William Daniel, Jr., The International Cultivator's Handbook Wingbow Press, 1974.

Dyer, Wayne, You'll See It When You Believe It, Morrow, 1989.

Ellis, Albert, "The Enlightened Atheist: An Interview with Albert Ellis," U*tne Reader* March-April 1997.

Flowers, Tom, M*arijuana Flower Forcing: Secrets of Designer Growing,* Flowers Publishing, 1997.
Flowers, Tom, M*arijuana Herbal Cookbook: Recipes for Recreation and Health,* Flowers Publishing, 1995.
Formukong, E. A., A. T. Evans, and F. J. Evans, "Analgesic and Anti-inflammatory Activity of Constitutents of Cannabis Sativa L." *Inflammation,* 12:4(1988).
Gascoigne, Bradley, and Julie Irwin, S*mart Ways to Stay Young and Healthy,* Ronin Publishing, Inc., 1992.
Gaskin, Stephen, C*annabis Spirituality,* High Times Books, 1996.
Gettman, John, "Marijuana and the Brain," H*igh Times,* March 1995.
Gieringer, Dale, "Marijuana Waterpipe/Vaporizer Study," MAPS, Spring 1996.
Gieringer, Dale, "Why Marijuana Smoke Harm Reduction?" MAPS, Spring 1996.
Gold, D., C*annabis Alchemy,* Ronin Publishing, Inc., 1989.
Gottlieb, Adam, T*he Art and Science of Cooking with Cannabis: The Most Effective Methods of Preparing Food and Drink with Marijuana, Hashish and Hash Oil,* Ronin Publishing, Inc., 1993.
Greenberg, J., J. H. Kuehnle, J. H. Mendelson, and J. G. Bernstein, "Effects of Marihuana Use on Body Weight and Caloric Intake in Humans," *Journal of Psychopharmacology* 49 (1976).
Griffith, H. Winter, *Complete Guide to Symptoms, Illness, and Surgery,* The Body Press, 1985.
Griffith, William, O*pium Poppy Garden: The Way of A Chinese Grower,* Ronin Publishing, 1993.
Grinspoon, Lester, and James B. Bakalar, "Marihuana as Medicine: A Plea for Reconsideration," J*ournal of the American Medical Association,* June 21, 1995.
Grinspoon, Lester, and James B. Bakalar, M*arihuana: The Forbidden Medicine,* Yale University Press, 1993.
Grinspoon, Lester, "Marihuana as Medicine," H*empWorld,* Fall 1996.
Grinspoon, Lester, "Marihuana," S*cientific American,* December 1969.
Hagman, George, "Stages of Change in Methadone Maintenance," J*ournal of Maintenance in the Addictions,* 1:1 (1997).
HempWorld Magazine, H*emp Pages: The Hemp Industry Sourcebook,* HempWorld, 1997.
Hepler, R. S., and I. M. Frank, "Marihuana Smoking and Intraocular Pressure," J*ournal of the American Medical Association* 217 (1971).
Herer, Jack, T*he Emporer Wears No Clothes: The Authoritative Historical Record of the Cannabis Plant, Hemp Prohibition, and How Marijuana Can Still Save the World,* Hemp/Queen of Clubs Publishing, 1990.
High Times Encyclopedia of Recreational Drugs, Stonehill Publishing Company, 1978.
Hofmann, Albert, L*SD: My Problem Child,* Jeremy P. Tarcher, Inc., 1983.
Hollister, Leo, "Marijuana and Immunity," *Journal of Psychoactive Drugs,* January-March 1988.
I Ching; or, Book of Changes, Wilhelm, Richard (translator), Third Edition, Princeton, 1967.
John-Roger, S*piritual Warrior,* Mandevile Press, Los Angeles, Ca, 1998.
Jones, Helen C., and Paul W. Lovinger, T*he Marijuana Question and Science's Search for an Answer,* Dodd, Mead, 1985.
Julien, Robert M., A *Primer of Drug Action: A Concise, Nontechnical Guide to the Actions, Uses, and Side Effects of Psychoactive Drugs,* 7th Edition, W. H. Freeman and Company, 1995.
Kassirer, Jerome P., "Federal Foolishness and Marijuana," N*ew England Journal of Medicine,* January 30, 1997.
Kerjci, Z., "On the Problem of Substances with Antibacterial Action: Cannabis Effect," C*asopis Lekaru Ceskych* 43 (1961).
Kershaw, Alex, "Medicine, Man," G*uardian* (UK), September 18, 1993.
Kong, Dolores, "Pot, a Balm to Some, Faces New Hurdle," *Boston Globe,* November 25, 1995.
Kotin, J., R. M. Post, and F. K. Goodwin, "Delta-9-tetrahydrocannabinol in Depressed Patients," A*rchives of General Psychiatry* 28 (1973).
Kramer, Peter D., *Listening to Prozac,* Viking, 1993.
Lancz, G., S. Specter, and H. K. Brown, "Suppressive Effect of Delta-9-tetrahydrocannabinol on Herpes Simplex Virus Infectivity in Vitro," P*roceedings of the Society for Experimental Biology and Medicine* 196 (1991).
Leary, Timothy, and R. U. Sirius, D*esign for Dying,* HarperSanFrancisco, 1997.
Leary, Timothy, H*igh Priest,* Ronin Pulbishing, 1996.
Leary, Timothy, P*sychedelic Prayers and Other Meditations,* Ronin Publishing, Inc., 1997.

Lorig, Kate, R.N., Dr.P.H., and James F. Fries, *The Arthritis Helpbook: A Tested Self-Management Program for Coping with Your Arthritis*, Revised Edition, Addison-Wesley, 1986.

Lovret, Fredrick J., *The Way And The Power: Secrets Of Japanese Strategy*, Paladin Press, Boulder, Co. 1987.

Ludlow, Fitzhugh, *The Hasheesh Eater*, Level Press, 1975.

Lyman, W. D., J. R. Sonnett, C. F. Brosnan, R. Elkin, and M. B. Bornstein, "Delta-9-tetrahydrocannabinol: A Novel Treatment for Experimental Autoimmune Encephalitis," *Journal of Neuroimmunology* 23 (1989).

Malec, J., R. F. Harvey, and J. J. Cayner, "Cannabis Effect on Spasticity in Spinal Cord Injury," *Archives of Physical and Medical Rehabilitation*, March 1982.

Mason, L. John, *Guide to Stress Reduction*, Celestial Arts, 1985.

Mathre, Mary Lynn, ed., *Cannabis in Medical Practice: A Legal, Historical, and Pharmacological Overview of the Therapeutic Uses of Marijuana*, McFarland and Company, 1997.

Mathre, Mary Lynn, "The Medicinal Uses of Marijuana," *Perspectives on Addictions Nursing*, June 1993.

Matsuda, L. A., S. J. Lolait, M. J. Brownstein, A. C. Young, and T. I. Bonner, "Structure of a Cannabinoid Receptor and Functional Expression of the Cloned cDNA," *Nature*, August 9, 1990.

Matthews, Dale A., David. B. Larson, and Constance P. Barry, *The Faith Factor: An Annotated Bibliography of Systematic Reviews and Clinical Research on Spiritual Subjects*. John Templeton Foundation, 1994.

Mattison, J. B., "*Cannabis indica* as an Anodyne and Hypnotic," *St. Louis Medical Surgical Journal* 61 (1891).

Maurer, M., V. Henn, A. Dittrich, and A. Hofmann, "Delta-9-tetrahydrocannabinol Shows Antispastic and Analgesic Effects in a Single Case Double-blind Trial," *European Archives of Psychiatry and Clinical Neuroscience* 240 (1990).

McGinnis, Alan Loy, *The Power of Optimism*, HarperPaperbacks, 1990.

Mechoulam, Raphael, ed., *Cannabinoids as Therapeutic Agents*, CRC Press, 1986.

Meinck, H. M., P. W. Schonle, and B. Conrad, "Effect of Cannabinoids on Spasticity and Ataxia in Multiple Sclerosis," *Journal of Neurology* 236 (1989).

Metcalf, C.W., and Roma Felible, *Lighten Up: Survival Skills For People Under Pressure*, Addison-Wesley, 1992.

Meyers, Frederick H., "Pharmacology of Marijuana: Just Another Sedative," presented at The Drug Policy Foundation's CME Seminar, November 13, 1992.

Mikuriya, Tod H., ed., *Marijuana: Medical Papers 1839-1972*, Medi-Comp Press, 1973.

Miller, Lyle H., and Alma Dell Smith, with Larry Rothstein, *The Stress Solution: An Action Plan to Manage the Stress in Your Life*, Pocket Books, 1993.

Milstein, S. L., K. MacCannell, G. Karr, and S. Clark, "Marijuana-produced Changes in Pain Tolerance: Experienced and Non-experienced Subjects," *International Pharmacopsychiatry* 10 (1975).

Mirken, Bruce, "Hope, Hype, and Survival: Do New Treatments Mean AIDS is No Longer Fatal—Or Have the Mass Media Blown It Yet Again?" *San Francisco Bay Times*, December 12, 1996.

Morgan, Roberta, *The Emotional Pharmacy: How Mood-Altering and Psychoactive Drugs Work*, The Body Press, 1988.

Morgenthaler, John, and Dan Joy, *Better Sex Through Chemistry: A Guide to the New Prosexual Drugs and Nutrients*, Smart Publications, 1995.

Murphy, Laura and Andrzej Bartke, eds., *Marijuana/Cannabinoids: Neurobiology and Neurophysiology*, CRC Press, 1992.

National Academy of Sciences, *Marijuana and Health*, National Academy Press, 1982.

Neufeldt, Victoria, Editor in Chief; Guralnik, David B., Editor in Chief Emeritus, *Webster's New World Dictionary of American English, Third College Edition*, Simon & Schuster, 1988.

Noyes, R., Jr., S. F. Brunk, D. A. Baram, and A. Canter, "Analgesic Effect of Delta-9-tetrahydrocannabinol," *Journal of Clinical Pharmacology*, February-March 1975.

Noyes, R., S. F. Brunk, D. H. Avery, and A. Canter, "The Analgesic Properties of Delta-9-tetrahydrocannabinol and Codeine," *Clinical Pharmacology and Therapeutics* 18 (1975).

O'Brien, Robert, and Sidney Cohen, *The Encyclopedia of Drug Abuse*, Facts on File, 1984.

Ott, Jonathan, *Pharmacotheon: Entheogenic Drugs, Their Plant Sources and History*, Natural Products Co., 1993.

Oxford Annotated Bible with the Apocrypha, Revised Standard Version, College Edition, Oxford University Press, 1965.

Palmer, Cynthia, and Michael Horowitz, eds. *Shaman Woman, Mainline Lady: Women's Writings on the Drug Experience*, Quill, 1982.

Pelletier, Kenneth R., *Mind as Healer, Mind As Slayer: A Holistic Approach to Preventing Stress Disorders*, Delta, 1977.

Pendell, Dale, *Pharmako/Poeia: Plant Powers, Poisons, and Herbcraft*, Mercury House, 1995.

Potter, Beverly A., and Sebastian Orfali, *Brain Boosters: Foods and Drugs That Make You Smarter*, Ronin Publishing, 1993.

Potter, Beverly A., *Finding a Path With A Heart: How To Go From Burnout To Bliss*, Ronin Publishing, 1995.

Potter, Beverly A., *Overcoming Job Burnout: How to Renew Your Enthusiasm for Work*, Ronin Publishing,1997.

Potter, Beverly A., *The Worrywart's Companion: Twenty-One Ways to Soothe Yourself and Worry Smart*, Wildcat Canyon Press, 1997.

Radcliffe, Anthony, Peter Ruch, Carol Forror Scott, Joe Cruse, *The Pharmer's Almanac: A Layman's Guide to Psychoactive Drugs*, Ballantine Books,1985.

Randall, R.C., ed., *Cancer Treatment and Marijuana Therapy* ("Marijuana, Medicine, and the Law" series), Galen Press, 1990.

Randall, R.C., ed., *Marijuana, Medicine, and the Law*, Galen Press, 1988.

Randall, R.C., ed., *Marijuana, Medicine, and the Law: Volume II*, Galen Press, 1989.

Randall, R.C., *Marijuana and AIDS: Pot, Politics, and PWAs in America*, Galen Press, 1991.

Rathbun, Mary, and Dennis Peron, *Brownie Mary's Cookbook and Dennis Peron's Recipe for Social Change*, Trail of Smoke Publishing Company, 1996.

Restak, Richard, "Brain by Design," *The Sciences*, September/October 1993.

Restak, Richard M., *Receptors*, Bantam Books, 1994.

Richardson, Jim, *Sinsemilla Marijuana Flowers*, And/Or Press, 1976.

Robinson, Rowan, *The Great Book of Hemp: The Complete Guide to the Environmental, Commericial, and Medicinal Uses of the World's Most Extraordinary Plant*, Park Street Press, 1996.

Roffman, Roger A. *Marijuana as Medicine*, Madrona Publishers, 1982.

Ronin Publishing Editors, *Fountains of Youth: How to Live Longer and Healthier*, Ronin Publishing, Inc., 1996.

Rosavear, John, *Pot: A Handbook of Marijauna*, The Citadel Press, 1967.

Rose, Jeanne, *Herbs and Things*, Workman Publishing Company, 1972.

Rosenthal, Ed, and Steve Kubby, *Why Marijuana Should Be Legal*, Thunder's Mouth Press, 1996.

Rosenthal, Ed, Dale Gieringer, and Tod Mikuriya, *Marijuana Medical Hnadbook: A Guide to Therapeutic Use*, Quick American Archives, 1997.

Rosenthal, Ed, *Marijuana Growing Tips*, Quick American Trading, 1986.

Rosenthal, Ed, William Logan, and Jeffrey Steinborn, *Marijuana, the Law, and You*, Quick American Archives, 1995.

Schultes, Richard Evans, and Albert Hofmann, *Plants of the Gods*, Healing Arts Press, 1992.

Seligman, Martin E. P., *Helplessness: On Depression, Development and Death*, Freeman and Company, 1975.

Seligman, Martin E. P., *What You Can Change And What You Can't: The Complete Guide To Successful Self-Improvement*, Fawcett Columbine, 1993.

Shulgin, Alexander T., *Controlled Substances: Chemical and Legal Guide to Federal Drug Laws*, Ronin Publishing, Inc., 1992.

Siegel, Ronald K., *Intoxication: Life in Pursuit of Artificial Paradise*, E. P. Dutton, 1989.

Smith, David E., ed., *The New Social Drug: Cultural, Medical, and Legal Perspectives on Marijuana*, Prentice-Hall, Inc., 1970.

Snyder, Solomon H., *Uses of Marijuana*, Oxford University Press, 1971.

Snyder, Solomon H., *Drugs and the Brain*, Scientific American Library Paperbacks, 1986.

Solomon, David, ed., *The Marihuana Papers*, Bobbs-Merrill, 1966.

Stafford, Peter, *Psychedelics Encyclopedia*, Third Expanded Edition, Ronin Publishing, Inc., 1992.

Starks, Michael, *Marijuana Chemistry: Genetics, Processing, and Potency*, Ronin Publishing, Inc., 1990.

Stockings, G. T., "A New Euphoriant for Depressive Mental States," *British Medical Journal* 1 (1947).

Storm, Daniel, *Marijuana Hydroponics: High-Tech Water Culture*, Ronin Publishing, Inc., 1987.

Strausbaugh, John, and Donald Blaise, eds., *The Drug User: Documents 1840-1960*, Blast/Dolphin, 1990.

Sumach, Alexander, *A Treasury of Hashish*, Stoneworks Publishing Company, 1976.

Tagami, Ty, "A Daughter's Pain," *Los Angleles Times*, January 2, 1995.

Tart, Charles T., *Altered States of Consciousness*, Doubleday and Company, 1972.

Tashkin, D. P., B. J. Shapiro, and I. A. Frank, "Acute Pulmonary Physiologic Effects of Smoked Marihuana and Oral Delta-9-tetrahydrocannabinol in Healthy Young Men," *New England Journal of Medicine* 289 (1973).

Tashkin, Donald P., Michael Simmons, and Virginia Clark, "Effect of Habitual Smoking of Marijuana Alone and with Tobacco on Nonspecific Airways Hyperreactivity," *Journal of Psychoactive Drugs*, January-March 1988.

Tashkin, D. P., S. Reiss, B. J. Shapiro, B. Calverese, J. L. Olson, and J. W. Lodge, "Bronchial Effects of Aerosolized Delta-9-THC in Healthy and Asthmatic Subjects," *American Review of Respiratory Disease* 115 (1987).

Thompson, L., and R. C. Proctor, "Parahexyl in the Treatment of Alcoholic and Drug Withdrawal Conditions," *North Carolina Journal of Medicine* 14:520 (1953).

Toklas, Alice B., *The Alice B. Toklas Cookbook*, Harper and Row, 1984.

Trebach, Arnold S., and Kevin B. Zeese, *Drug Prohibition and the Conscience of Nations*, The Drug Policy Foundation, 1990.

Vinceguerra, T. Moore, and E. Brennan, "Inhalation Marijuana as an Anti-emetic for Cancer Chemotherapy," *New York State Journal of Medicine*, October 1988.

Volfe, Z., A. Dilansky, and I. Nathan, "Cannabinoids Block Release of Serotonin from Platelets Induced by Plasma from Migraine Patients," *International Journal of Clinical Pharmacological Research*, 4 (1985).

Wasson, R. Gordon, Stella Kamrisch, Jonathon Ott, and Carl A. P. Ruck, *Persephone's Quest: Entheogens and the Origins of Religion*, Yale University Press, 1986.

Weil, Andrew, and Winifred Rosen, *Chocolate to Morphine: Understanding Mind-Active Drugs*, Houghton Mifflin, 1983.

Weil, Andrew, *Health and Healing*, Houghton Mifflin Company, 1988.

Weil, Andrew, *The Natural Mind: A New Way of Looking at Drugs and the Higher Consciousness*, Houghton Mifflin, 1972.

Weil, Andrew, *Spontaneous Healing: How to Discover and Enhance Your Body's Natural Ability to Maintain and Heal Itself*, Alfred A. Knopf, 1995.

Weil, Andrew, *Natural Health, Natural Medicine: A Comprehensive Manual for Wellness and Self-Care*, Houghton Mifflin, 1990.

Woodward, Kenneth L., "Is God Listening?" *Newsweek*, March 31, 1997.

Zuardi, A. W., I. Shirakawa, E. Finkelbarb, and I. G. Karniol, "Action of Cannabidiol on the Anxiety and Other Effects Produced by Delta-9-THC in Normal Subjects," *Psychopharmacology* 76 (1976).

INDEX